KIDNEY DISEASE
DIET FOR STAGE 3
cookbook

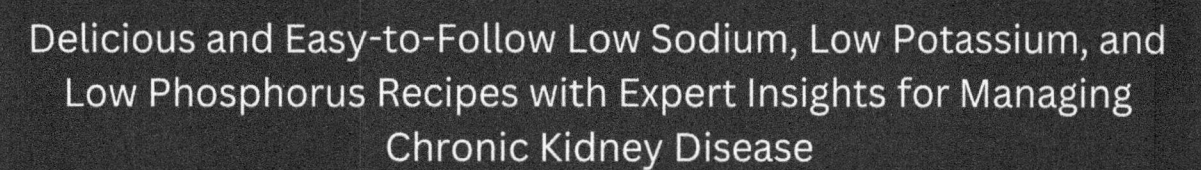

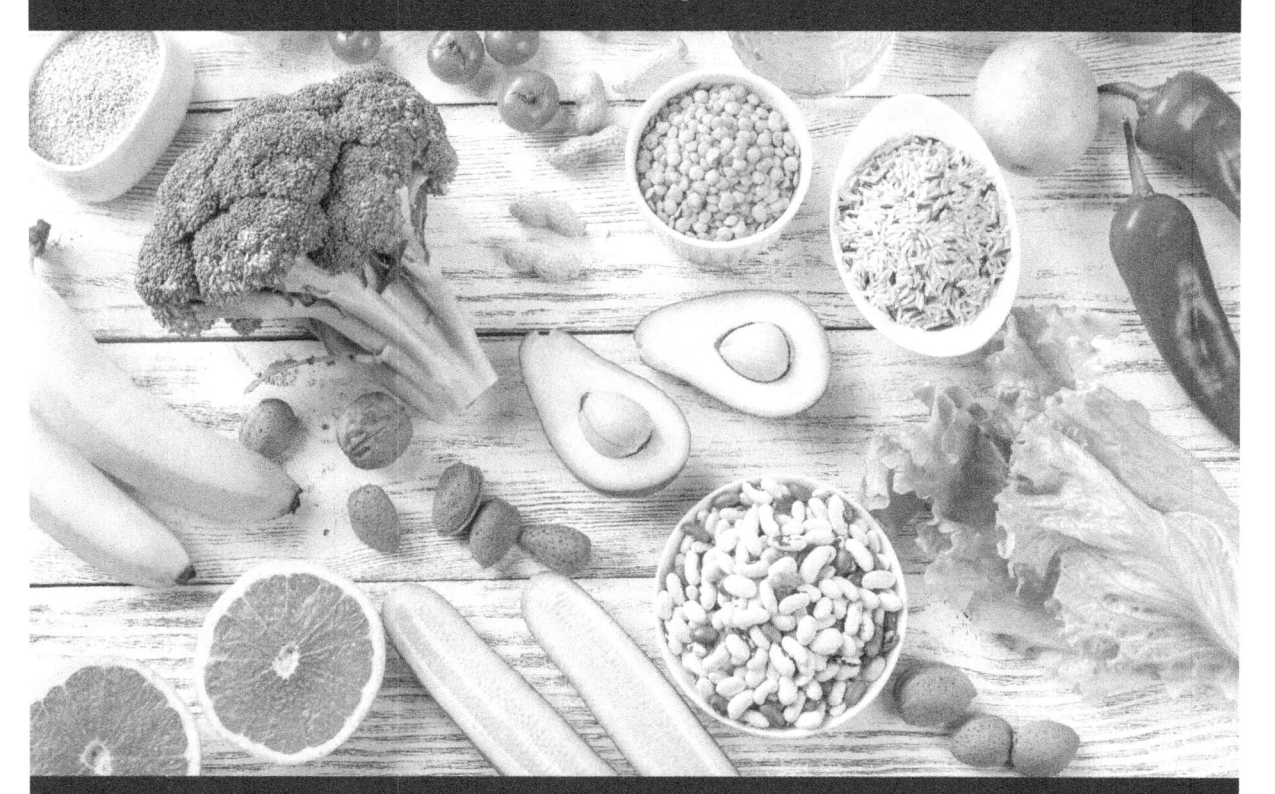

Delicious and Easy-to-Follow Low Sodium, Low Potassium, and Low Phosphorus Recipes with Expert Insights for Managing Chronic Kidney Disease

Emily M. Wilson

Copyright © 2023 Dr. Emily M. Wilson

All rights reserved.

No part of this publication may be reproduced, distributed, or transmitted in any form or by any means, including photocopying, recording, or other electronic or mechanical methods, without the prior written permission of the publisher, except in the case of brief quotations embodied in critical reviews and certain other noncommercial uses permitted by copyright law.

PREFACE

THE STORY THAT INSPIRED THE CREATION OF THIS BOOK

Halle had always been the kind of woman who could handle anything life threw at her. At fifty-two, she was the definition of resilience, a mother of two, a loving wife, and a career woman who juggled her responsibilities with grace. But sometimes, life has a way of humbling even the strongest among us.

One brisk autumn morning, Halle woke up feeling unusually fatigued. The energy that used to propel her through her day had waned, leaving her listless and drained. It was a feeling she couldn't quite shake off. Day by day, the fatigue persisted, as did the constant gnawing sensation in her bones. Her once-radiant skin took on a pallor that concerned her family and friends.

As weeks turned into months, the symptoms intensified. Swelling, or edema as she would soon learn, began to manifest in her legs and ankles. It was a swelling that seemed to mock her, a reminder that her body was no longer functioning as it should. Halle's visits to the bathroom increased in frequency, and she noticed that her urine had become darker and frothier than usual.

Afraid and unsure of what was happening to her body, Halle decided to seek medical advice. Her family doctor, a kind and empathetic man, listened attentively as she recounted her symptoms. After a thorough examination and a battery of tests, the diagnosis was delivered with a solemnity that sent shivers down her spine: Stage 3 Kidney Disease, also known as Chronic Kidney Disease (CKD).

Halle sat in that sterile examination room, the weight of the diagnosis bearing down on her shoulders like a leaden cloak. Chronic Kidney Disease, the doctor explained, meant that her kidneys were no longer functioning at full capacity. The glomerular filtration rate (GFR), a measure of kidney function, had fallen below 60 milliliters per minute. Her kidneys were struggling to filter waste and excess fluids from her blood, leading to the symptoms she had been experiencing.

Tears welled up in Halle's eyes as she contemplated what this diagnosis meant for her life. It wasn't just the physical discomfort; it was the looming uncertainty, the fear of what lay ahead.

She thought of her family, her husband, and her children, and the prospect of dialysis or even a kidney transplant seemed overwhelming.

However, her doctor, aware of her despair, offered a glimmer of hope. He explained that while CKD was a serious condition, its progression could be slowed, and sometimes even reversed, with the right interventions. He emphasized the pivotal role that diet plays in managing CKD.

Leaving the clinic with a heavy heart but newfound determination, Halle embarked on a journey to regain control of her life. She educated herself about CKD, pouring over medical literature and consulting with specialists. She learned that a kidney-friendly diet could alleviate the strain on her kidneys and potentially improve their function.

The importance of diet in managing CKD became her guiding light. Halle discovered that a kidney-friendly diet wasn't about deprivation, but about making thoughtful choices that supported her kidney health. It was about understanding how certain foods could exacerbate the disease and how others could be her allies in the battle against it.

With the support of a registered dietitian, Halle revamped her eating habits. She learned to monitor her sodium intake, as excessive salt could lead to fluid retention and high blood pressure. By reducing her sodium consumption and embracing herbs and spices as flavorful alternatives, she regained some control over her edema.

Protein was another critical aspect of her diet. Halle discovered that excessive protein intake could strain her kidneys, so she worked with her dietitian to find the right balance. High-quality sources of protein, such as lean poultry and fish, replaced some of the red meat in her meals. Her dietitian also helped her calculate her daily protein needs, ensuring she received enough to maintain her strength while sparing her kidneys from undue stress.

Phosphorus and potassium management became her daily mission. She learned that elevated levels of these minerals could wreak havoc on her already weakened kidneys. Halle diligently avoided high-phosphorus foods like processed meats and colas, opting instead for fresh fruits and vegetables that were lower in potassium. She also took phosphate binders as prescribed by her healthcare team to help control phosphorus levels.

Staying hydrated was crucial, but she had to be mindful of her fluid intake. Halle learned that excessive fluids could lead to swelling and high blood pressure, so she carefully measured her daily fluid intake and followed her doctor's recommendations.

As Halle embraced these dietary changes, she found herself experiencing small victories. Her energy levels slowly improved, and the relentless fatigue began to lift. The swelling in her legs and ankles gradually subsided, and her skin regained its healthy glow. The emotional toll of her diagnosis began to ease as well, as she felt more in control of her health and her future.

Months turned into years, and Halle continued to prioritize her kidney-friendly diet. Regular check-ups with her healthcare team showed signs of improvement in her kidney function. Her GFR began to inch its way back up, signaling that her kidneys were finding some respite. Halle's journey wasn't without its challenges, but she faced them with determination and the unwavering support of her loved ones.

As Halle reflects on her journey, she knows that her story is one of hope. It's a testament to the power of knowledge, resilience, and the pivotal role that diet can play in managing Chronic Kidney Disease. It's a story that she hopes will inspire others facing similar challenges to take control of their health and embrace the healing potential of a kidney-friendly diet.

In the pages that follow, we will explore the world of kidney-friendly nutrition together. We will delve into delicious recipes and meal plans designed to support kidney health, offering a lifeline to those navigating the complex terrain of Stage 3 Kidney Disease. Halle's story is just the beginning, and the cookbook that follows is a roadmap to a healthier, brighter future.

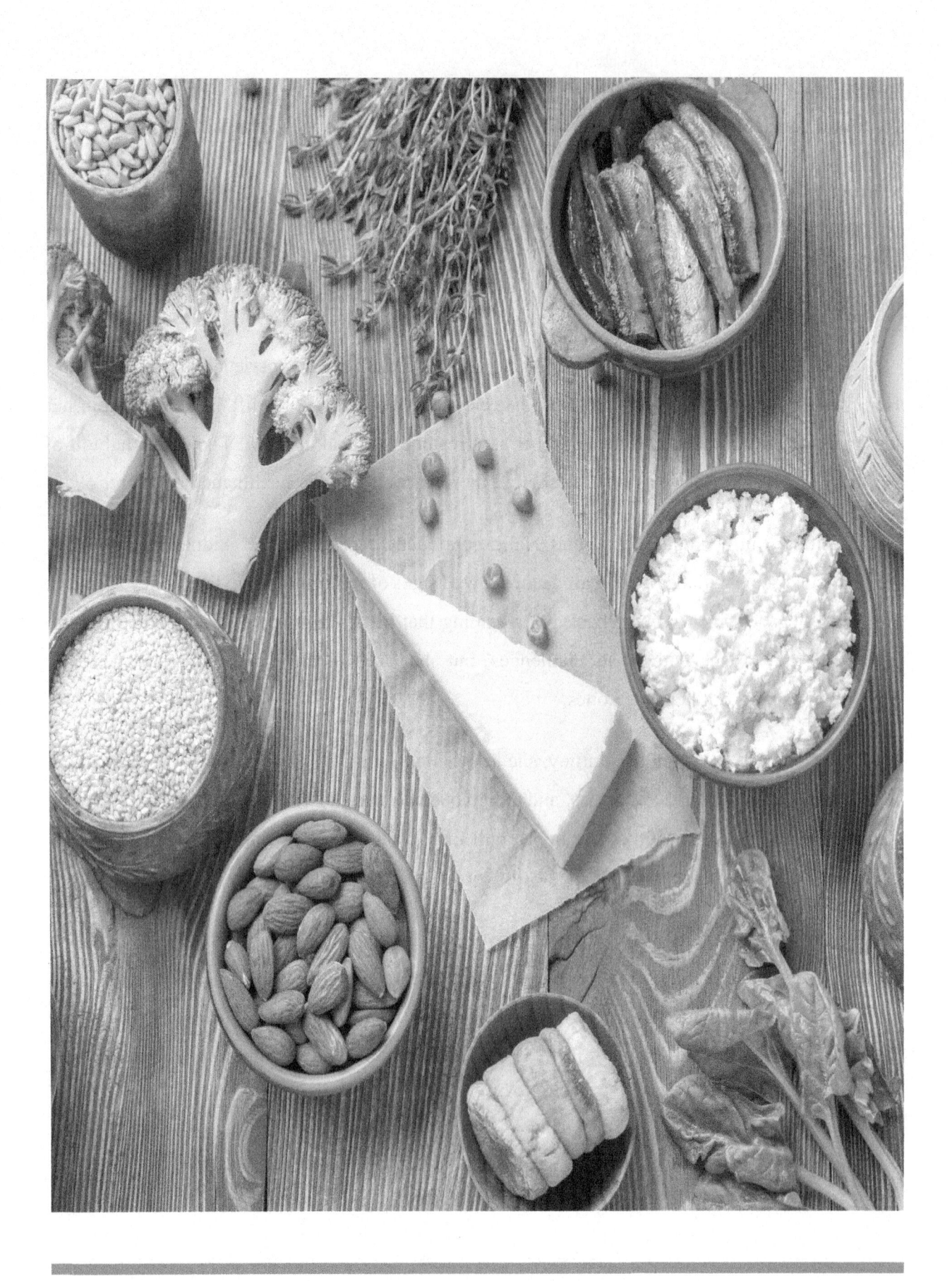

Contents

INTRODUCTION 11

UNDERSTANDING KIDNEY DISEASE 11

COMMON CAUSES OF KIDNEY DISEASE 11

SYMPTOMS AND DIAGNOSIS 12

KIDNEY DISEASE RISK FACTORS 13

THE ROLES OF NUTRITION IN MANAGING STAGE 3 KIDNEY DISEASE 14

CHAPTER ONE: RECIPES 17

BREAKFAST RECIPES 17

    Creamy Oatmeal with Blueberries 17

    Egg White and Vegetable Scramble 18

    Greek Yogurt Parfait 19

    Cottage Cheese and Peach Bowl 20

    Quinoa Breakfast Bowl 21

    Sweet Potato Hash 22

    Baked Apple with Cinnamon 23

    Rice Cake with Peanut Butter and Banana 24

    Millet Breakfast Bowl 25

    Vegetable and Cheese Breakfast Quesadilla 26

LUNCH RECIPES 27

    Grilled Chicken Salad 27

    White Bean and Vegetable Soup 28

    Tuna Salad Lettuce Wraps 29

    Turkey and Avocado Wrap 30

    Lemon Herb Baked Salmon 31

    Mediterranean Chickpea Salad 32

    Vegetable and Brown Rice Stir-Fry 33

    Lentil and Spinach Soup 34

Tofu and Vegetable Stir-Fry 35

Lemon Dill Shrimp Skewers 36

DINNER RECIPES 37

Stuffed Bell Peppers 37

Lemon Garlic Shrimp and Asparagus 38

Cauliflower and Spinach Curry 39

Mushroom and Quinoa Stuffed Acorn Squash 40

Lemon Herb Baked Cod 41

Spaghetti Squash Primavera 42

Lentil and Sweet Potato Curry 43

Baked Eggplant Parmesan 44

Grilled Portobello Mushrooms with Balsamic Glaze 45

Quinoa and Black Bean Stuffed Peppers 46

SNACKS AND APPETIZERS 47

Hummus and Veggie Platter 47

Cucumber and Greek Yogurt Dip 47

Stuffed Celery Sticks 48

Baked Sweet Potato Fries 49

Roasted Chickpeas 50

Mozzarella and Tomato Skewers 51

Avocado and Tomato Salsa 51

Spinach and Artichoke Dip (Low Sodium Version) 52

Baked Zucchini Chips 53

Sliced Apple with Almond Butter 54

MAIN COURSES (INCLUDING VEGETARIAN OPTIONS) 55

Grilled Lemon Herb Chicken 55

Eggplant Parmesan (Vegetarian) 56

Lentil and Vegetable Stir-Fry (Vegetarian) 57

Baked Salmon with Dill Sauce 58

Spinach and Mushroom Risotto (Vegetarian) 59

Turkey and Vegetable Stir-Fry 60

Sweet Potato and Black Bean Tacos (Vegetarian) 61

Lemon Garlic Roasted Tofu and Vegetables (Vegan) 62

SOUPS AND SALADS RECIPES 63

Creamy Cauliflower Soup 63

Roasted Red Pepper and Lentil Soup 64

Greek Quinoa Salad 65

Chicken and Rice Soup 66

Tuna Salad 67

Minestrone Soup 68

Quinoa and Black Bean Soup 69

Spinach and Strawberry Salad 71

Butternut Squash Soup 72

Chickpea and Avocado Salad 73

Tomato Basil Soup 74

Cucumber and Dill Salad 75

DESSERTS AND TREATS 77

Banana Ice Cream 77

Baked Apples 77

Rice Pudding 78

Chocolate Avocado Mousse 79

Oatmeal Raisin Cookies 80

Berry Parfait 81

Pineapple Sorbet 82

Lemon Bars 83

Frozen Yogurt Bites 84

Chocolate-Covered Strawberries 85

BEVERAGES 87

HERBAL TEAS FOR KIDNEY SUPPORT 87

Dandelion Root Tea 87

Nettle Leaf Tea 88
Hibiscus Tea 89
Ginger Tea 90
Parsley Tea 91

LOW POTASSIUM-INFUSED WATER 92
Cucumber and Mint Infused Water 92
Lemon and Lime Infused Water 93
Berry Blast Infused Water 94
Peach and Basil Infused Water 95

HOMEMADE ELECTROLYTE DRINKS 96
DIY Electrolyte Solution 96
Green Tea Electrolyte Cooler 97
Pineapple Coconut Electrolyte Smoothie 98
Watermelon and Mint Electrolyte Refresher 99
Coconut Water Electrolyte Drink 100
Watermelon Electrolyte Cooler 101

CHAPTER TWO: 30-DAY MEAL PLAN AND GROCERY SHOPPING GUIDE 103

GROCERY SHOPPING GUIDE 107

CONCLUSION 111

MEAL PLANNING JOURNAL **113**

INTRODUCTION

UNDERSTANDING KIDNEY DISEASE

Kidney disease, also known as renal disease or nephropathy, is a complex and frequently progressive medical condition that affects the kidneys' ability to filter waste and excess fluids from the blood, maintain electrolyte balance, and regulate blood pressure. Understanding kidney disease is crucial for early detection, therapy, and general health preservation.

COMMON CAUSES OF KIDNEY DISEASE

Kidney disease can be caused by a number of reasons, some of which are common in today's society. Understanding the causes is important for early detection and prevention. Here are some of the most common causes of kidney disease:

1. **Hypertension (High Blood Pressure):** Hypertension is a major cause of renal disease. The kidneys play an important role in blood pressure regulation. When blood pressure is consistently high, it can damage the small blood vessels in the kidneys, reducing their ability to filter waste and excess fluids from the body.
2. **Diabetes:** Diabetes, both type 1 and type 2, is another major cause of kidney disease. High blood sugar levels can damage the blood vessels in the kidneys, eventually causing kidney disease. Diabetic kidney disease, commonly known as diabetic nephropathy, is a common diabetic complication.
3. **Glomerulonephritis:** Glomerulonephritis is a group of diseases that cause inflammation and injury to the glomeruli, which are small units within the kidneys that filter blood. Infections, immune system diseases, and genetic factors can all contribute to glomerulonephritis.
4. **Polycystic Kidney Disease (PKD):** PKD is a genetic disorder that causes the kidneys to develop many fluid-filled cysts. These cysts can eventually replace healthy kidney tissue, limiting kidney function. In adults, PKD is the main cause of kidney failure.

5. **Urinary Tract Infections (UTIs):** Recurrent or untreated UTIs can progress to kidney infections, which can cause kidney damage if severe or untreated. Kidney infections are a common but preventable cause of kidney disease.

SYMPTOMS AND DIAGNOSIS

Kidney disease symptoms can vary based on the stage and its cause. Kidney disease can be asymptomatic in the early stages, making it difficult to detect. However, when the condition worsens, the following symptoms may become evident:

1. **Fatigue:** Excessive tiredness or weakness might be an early indicator of kidney disease. As the kidneys work to filter waste and maintain normal balance, anemia can develop, causing fatigue.
2. **Urinary Changes:** Kidney disease can cause changes in urine flow and appearance. Foamy pee, frequent urination, especially at night (Nocturia), and difficulty or pain during urinating are all symptoms.
3. **Swelling:** Kidney disease can cause fluid retention, resulting in swelling around the ankles, legs, and eyes. This is known as edema, and it is a common indication of kidney dysfunction.
4. **High Blood Pressure:** High blood pressure can be both a cause and a symptom of kidney disease if it is not controlled. Blood pressure monitoring is critical in the treatment of kidney disease.
5. **Blood in Urine (Hematuria):** The presence of blood in the urine can suggest kidney damage or the presence of kidney stones. It is not usually obvious, but a urine test can reveal it.
6. **Protein in Urine (Proteinuria):** Healthy kidneys filter waste while retaining vital proteins in the blood circulation. Proteinuria occurs when the kidneys are compromised and allow excess protein to escape into the urine.

DIAGNOSIS

A medical history, physical examination, and laboratory tests are commonly used to diagnose renal disease. Among the most important diagnostic tests are:

- **Blood Tests:** These determine the levels of creatinine and blood urea nitrogen (BUN), which show how well the kidneys filter waste from the blood. Abnormal levels can suggest renal disease.
- Urine Tests: A urinalysis can identify protein, blood, or other abnormalities in the urine.
- **Imaging:** Ultrasounds, CT scans, and MRIs can be performed to visualize the kidneys and identify any structural abnormalities or cysts.
- **Kidney Biopsy:** A kidney biopsy may be required in some circumstances to diagnose the source of kidney disease, particularly if glomerulonephritis or other specific disorders are suspected.

KIDNEY DISEASE RISK FACTORS

Several risk factors increase a person's chances of having kidney disease:

1. **Diabetes:** Diabetics, particularly those with poorly regulated blood sugar levels, are more likely to develop renal damage.
2. **Hypertension:** High blood pressure can cause kidney damage over time, increasing the risk of kidney disease.
3. **Family History:** A family history of kidney disease, especially polycystic kidney disease, can raise the risk.
4. **Age:** The risk of kidney disease rises with age, particularly after the age of 50.
5. **Heart Disease:** Heart conditions, such as heart failure and coronary artery disease, can aggravate kidney problems.
6. **Obesity:** Obesity is a risk factor for diabetes and hypertension, both of which are major causes of kidney disease.
7. **Smoking:** Tobacco use can harm blood vessels, particularly those in the kidneys, impairing their ability to function properly.

8. **Certain Medications:** Long-term use of some medications, such as nonsteroidal anti-inflammatory drugs (NSAIDs), can affect the kidneys.
9. **Infections:** If left untreated, recurrent urinary tract infections (UTIs) and kidney infections can cause kidney damage.
10. **Kidney Stones:** Having kidney stones on a regular basis can increase the risk of kidney damage.

Understanding the common causes, symptoms, and risk factors for kidney disease is crucial for early detection and preventive therapy. Regular check-ups and a healthy lifestyle can help reduce these risks and enhance kidney health. If you have any worries about your kidney health or observe any strange symptoms, it is critical that you visit with a healthcare specialist for an accurate diagnosis and treatment.

THE ROLES OF NUTRITION IN MANAGING STAGE 3 KIDNEY DISEASE

Nutrition plays an important role in the management of Stage 3 Kidney Disease, also known as Chronic Kidney Disease (CKD). At this point, kidney function is significantly reduced, and a kidney-friendly diet becomes critical for delaying disease progression and enhancing general well-being. The following are the key roles that diet plays in the management of Stage 3 CKD:

1. **Stress Reduction for the Kidneys:** A kidney-friendly diet seeks to lessen the stress on the kidneys by controlling the intake of certain nutrients. Limiting protein consumption, particularly from animal sources, is important because too much protein can strain the kidneys. By adjusting protein consumption, the kidneys can better manage waste products.
2. **Electrolyte Balance:** Kidney disease may disrupt the body's electrolyte balance, resulting in potassium, phosphorus, and sodium abnormalities. Through dietary changes, nutrition can help manage these electrolytes. Limiting potassium-rich foods, for example, can help prevent harmful surges in blood potassium levels.
3. **Blood Pressure Control:** Hypertension is a typical consequence of kidney disease. Nutrition is important in blood pressure management, with a focus on lowering sodium

intake. A low-sodium diet reduces fluid retention and high blood pressure, reducing the stress on the kidneys.

4. **Monitoring Fluid Intake:** The kidneys control fluid balance in the body. To avoid fluid overload, people with Stage 3 CKD may need to limit their fluid intake. A kidney-friendly diet outlines how to manage daily fluid intake to avoid edema and swelling.

5. **Maintaining appropriate Nutrition:** Regardless of dietary restrictions, maintaining appropriate nutrition is critical to preventing malnutrition. A well-balanced kidney diet provides enough calories, vitamins, and minerals while limiting harmful substances.

6. **Prevention of Further Complications:** Nutrition can help prevent complications linked with kidney disease, such as anemia. Iron-rich meals and proper protein management can help battle anemia, which is a prevalent problem in people with CKD.

7. **Enhancing Quality of Life:** A well-managed kidney diet can improve overall quality of life by reducing symptoms like fatigue, swelling, and fluid imbalances. It can also help maintain energy levels and support mental well-being.

8. **Slowing Disease Progression:** While nutrition cannot cure kidney disease, it can help slow down its progression. Individuals with Stage 3 CKD can delay the need for dialysis or kidney transplantation by following dietary advice and maintaining kidney function for an extended period.

Individuals with Stage 3 Kidney Disease must collaborate closely with healthcare practitioners and qualified dietitians to create a specific nutrition plan. Individual demands, stage of renal disease, comorbidities (such as diabetes or hypertension), and dietary preferences are all taken into account in these regimens. Individuals can better manage their kidney disease, enhance their quality of life, and potentially prevent the progression to more severe stages of CKD by combining dietary changes and medicinal therapy.

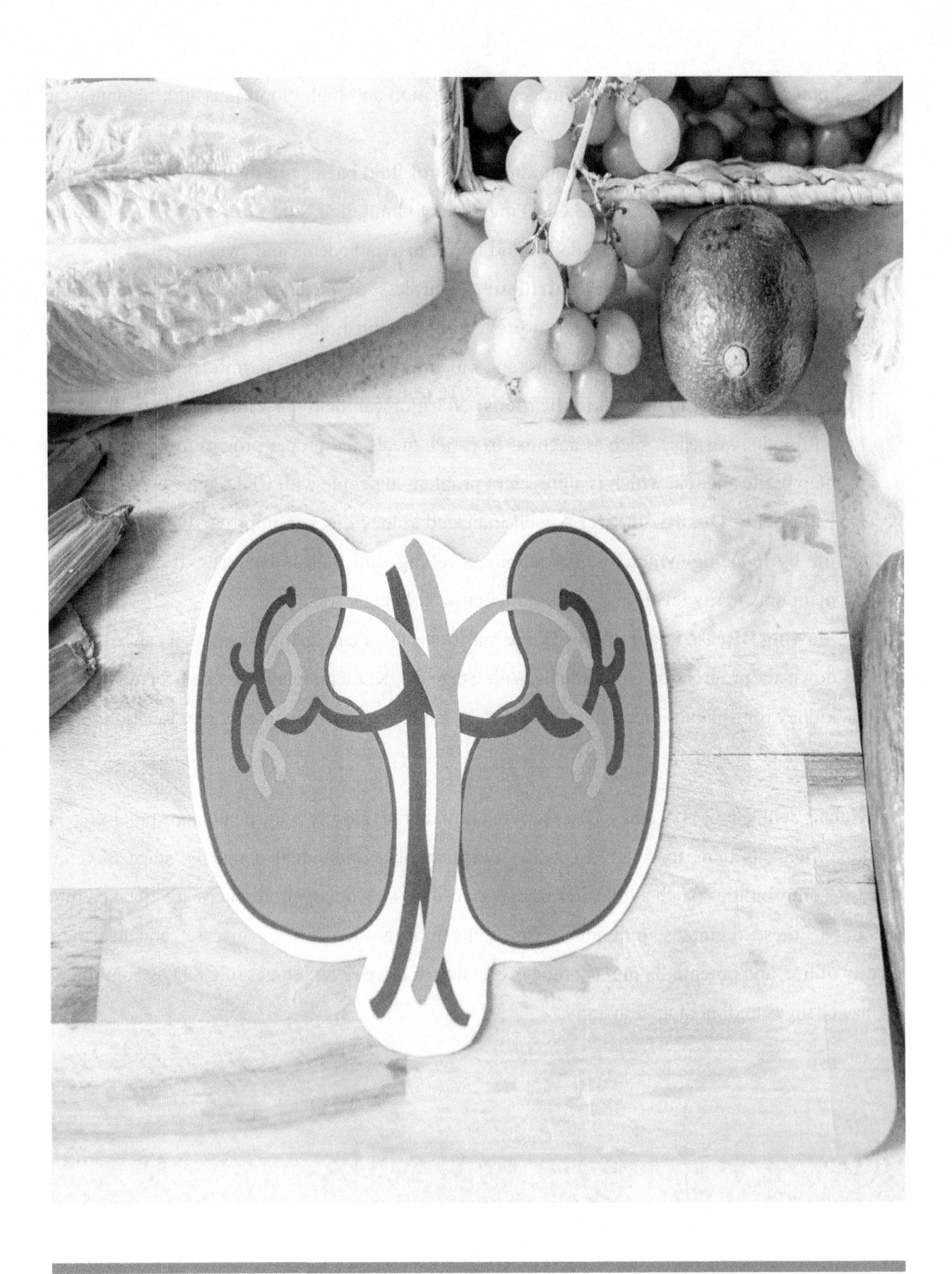

CHAPTER ONE: RECIPES

BREAKFAST RECIPES

CREAMY OATMEAL WITH BLUEBERRIES

Benefit: High fiber content aids digestion and keeps you feeling full.

- Prep/Cook Time: 15 minutes
- Servings: 2

Ingredients:

- 1 cup of steel-cut oats
- 2 cups of water
- 1/2 cup of fresh blueberries
- 1 tablespoon of honey (optional)
- 2 tablespoons of chopped walnuts (optional)

Cooking Instructions:

1. In a saucepan, bring water to a boil.
2. Add oats and reduce heat to a simmer. Cook for about 10 minutes or until creamy.
3. Serve hot, topped with blueberries and a drizzle of honey. Sprinkle with chopped walnuts if desired.

Nutritional Information (per serving):

- Calories: 250
- Protein: 6g
- Carbohydrates: 45g
- Fiber: 7g
- Potassium: 160mg

EGG WHITE AND VEGETABLE SCRAMBLE

Benefit: Low in phosphorus and potassium, high in protein.

- Prep/Cook Time: 15 minutes
- Servings: 2

Ingredients:

- 4 egg whites
- 1/4 cup of diced bell peppers
- 1/4 cup of diced onions
- 1/4 cup of diced tomatoes
- 1/4 cup of chopped spinach
- Salt and pepper to taste

Cooking Instructions:

1. Heat a non-stick skillet over medium heat.
2. Spray with cooking spray or a small amount of oil.
3. Add the vegetables and sauté until they soften.
4. Pour in the egg whites and cook, stirring gently, until they are set.
5. Season with salt and pepper.

Nutritional Information (per serving):

- Calories: 70
- Protein: 14g
- Carbohydrates: 4g
- Fiber: 1g
- Potassium: 200mg

GREEK YOGURT PARFAIT

Benefit: High in protein and probiotics for gut health.

- Prep/Cook Time: 10 minutes
- Servings: 2

Ingredients:

- 1 cup of low-fat Greek yogurt
- 1/2 cup of sliced strawberries
- 1/4 cup of granola (low sodium)
- 1 tablespoon of honey (optional)

Cooking Instructions:

1. In two serving glasses or bowls, layer Greek yogurt, strawberries, and granola.
2. Drizzle honey over the top if desired.

Nutritional Information (per serving):

- Calories: 180
- Protein: 12g
- Carbohydrates: 28g
- Fiber: 3g
- Potassium: 200mg

COTTAGE CHEESE AND PEACH BOWL

Benefit: Rich in protein and low in potassium.

- Prep/Cook Time: 5 minutes
- Servings: 1

Ingredients:

- 1/2 cup of low-fat cottage cheese
- 1 fresh peach, sliced
- 1/4 teaspoon of cinnamon
- 1 teaspoon of honey (optional)

Cooking Instructions:

1. In a bowl, add the cottage cheese.
2. Top with peach slices and sprinkle with cinnamon.
3. Drizzle with honey if desired.

Nutritional Information (per serving):

- Calories: 180
- Protein: 14g
- Carbohydrates: 30g
- Fiber: 3g
- Potassium: 290mg

QUINOA BREAKFAST BOWL

Benefit: High in protein, fiber, and essential nutrients.

- Prep/Cook Time: 20 minutes
- Servings: 2

Ingredients:

- 1 cup of cooked quinoa
- 1/2 cup of sliced bananas
- 1/4 cup of chopped almonds
- 1/4 teaspoon of cinnamon
- 1/2 cup of low-fat milk or milk alternative

Cooking Instructions:

1. In a bowl, combine quinoa, sliced bananas, and chopped almonds.
2. Sprinkle with cinnamon and pour in milk.
3. Stir and serve.

Nutritional Information (per serving):

- Calories: 300
- Protein: 10g
- Carbohydrates: 48g
- Fiber: 6g
- Potassium: 360mg

SWEET POTATO HASH

Benefit: Low in phosphorus and potassium, high in fiber.

- Prep/Cook Time: 30 minutes
- Servings: 2

Ingredients:

- 2 cups of diced sweet potatoes
- 1/2 cup of diced onions
- 1/2 cup of diced red bell peppers
- 1/2 cup of chopped spinach
- 2 teaspoons of olive oil
- Salt and pepper to taste

Cooking Instructions:

1. Heat olive oil in a skillet over medium-high heat.
2. Add sweet potatoes and sauté until they start to brown and become tender.
3. Add onions and bell peppers, and sauté until they soften.
4. Stir in chopped spinach and cook until wilted.
5. Season with salt and pepper.

Nutritional Information (per serving):

- Calories: 200
- Protein: 3g
- Carbohydrates: 35g
- Fiber: 5g
- Potassium: 300mg

BAKED APPLE WITH CINNAMON

Benefit: Low in sodium and potassium, high in fiber and antioxidants.

- Prep/Cook Time: 40 minutes
- Servings: 2

Ingredients:

- 2 apples, cored
- 1/2 teaspoon of cinnamon
- 1 tablespoon of chopped walnuts (optional)
- 1 tablespoon of raisins (optional)

Cooking Instructions:

1. Preheat the oven to 375°F (190°C).
2. Sprinkle the cored apples with cinnamon and place them in a baking dish.
3. Bake for 30-40 minutes until apples are tender.
4. Serve with chopped walnuts and raisins if desired.

Nutritional Information (per serving):

- Calories: 100
- Protein: 1g
- Carbohydrates: 25g
- Fiber: 5g
- Potassium: 190mg

RICE CAKE WITH PEANUT BUTTER AND BANANA

Benefit: Quick and easy, low in phosphorus and potassium.

- Prep/Cook Time: 5 minutes
- Servings: 1

Ingredients:

- 1 rice cake
- 1 tablespoon of peanut butter (low sodium)
- 1/2 banana, sliced

Cooking Instructions:

1. Spread peanut butter on the rice cake.
2. Top with banana slices.

Nutritional Information (per serving):

- Calories: 180
- Protein: 4g
- Carbohydrates: 28g
- Fiber: 3g
- Potassium: 180mg

MILLET BREAKFAST BOWL

Benefit: Gluten-free, high in protein and fiber.

- Prep/Cook Time: 25 minutes
- Servings: 2

Ingredients:

- 1 cup of cooked millet
- 1/2 cup of diced mango
- 2 tablespoons of chopped almonds
- 1/4 teaspoon of vanilla extract
- 1/2 cup of low-fat milk or milk alternative

Cooking Instructions:

1. In a bowl, combine cooked millet, diced mango, and chopped almonds.
2. Add vanilla extract and pour in milk.
3. Stir and serve.

Nutritional Information (per serving):

- Calories: 250
- Protein: 7g
- Carbohydrates: 44g
- Fiber: 5g
- Potassium: 220mg

VEGETABLE AND CHEESE BREAKFAST QUESADILLA

Benefit: High in protein, customizable with kidney-friendly vegetables.

- Prep/Cook Time: 20 minutes
- Servings: 2

Ingredients:

- 2 whole-wheat tortillas (low sodium)
- 4 egg whites
- 1/2 cup of diced bell peppers
- 1/4 cup of diced onions
- 1/4 cup of low-sodium shredded cheese
- Salt and pepper to taste

Cooking Instructions:

1. In a bowl, beat the egg whites and season with salt and pepper.
2. In a non-stick skillet, cook the egg whites over medium heat until set.
3. Place one tortilla in the skillet and layer with half of the cooked egg whites, diced vegetables, and shredded cheese.
4. Top with the second tortilla and cook until the cheese melts and the quesadilla is golden brown on both sides.
5. Cut into wedges and serve.

Nutritional Information (per serving):

- Calories: 270
- Protein: 15g
- Carbohydrates: 30g
- Fiber: 5g
- Potassium: 280mg

LUNCH RECIPES

GRILLED CHICKEN SALAD

Benefit: High in protein, low in sodium and potassium.

- Prep/Cook Time: 30 minutes
- Servings: 2

Ingredients:

- 2 boneless, skinless chicken breasts (4 ounces each)
- 4 cups of mixed salad greens
- 1/2 cucumber, sliced
- 1/2 cup of cherry tomatoes, halved
- 2 tablespoons of balsamic vinaigrette dressing (low sodium)
- Salt and pepper to taste

Cooking Instructions:

1. Season chicken breasts with salt and pepper.
2. Grill the chicken until cooked through, about 6-8 minutes per side.
3. Slice the grilled chicken.
4. In a large bowl, combine salad greens, cucumber, and cherry tomatoes.
5. Top with sliced chicken and drizzle with balsamic vinaigrette.

Nutritional Information (per serving):

- Calories: 220
- Protein: 26g
- Carbohydrates: 10g
- Fiber: 3g
- Potassium: 330mg

WHITE BEAN AND VEGETABLE SOUP

Benefit: Low in sodium and potassium, high in fiber.

- Prep/Cook Time: 40 minutes
- Servings: 4

Ingredients:

- 1 can (15 ounces) of low-sodium white beans, drained and rinsed
- 1 cup of diced carrots
- 1 cup of diced celery
- 1 cup of diced zucchini
- 1/2 cup of diced onions
- 4 cups of low-sodium vegetable broth
- 1 teaspoon of dried thyme
- Salt and pepper to taste

Cooking Instructions:

1. In a large pot, sauté onions, carrots, celery, and zucchini until softened.
2. Add white beans, vegetable broth, thyme, salt, and pepper.
3. Simmer for 20-25 minutes.
4. Serve hot.

Nutritional Information (per serving):

- Calories: 150
- Protein: 7g
- Carbohydrates: 28g
- Fiber: 7g
- Potassium: 380mg

TUNA SALAD LETTUCE WRAPS

Benefit: High in protein, low in sodium and potassium.

- Prep/Cook Time: 15 minutes
- Servings: 2

Ingredients:

- 1 can (5 ounces) of low-sodium tuna, drained
- 1/4 cup of diced celery
- 1/4 cup of diced red bell peppers
- 2 tablespoons of light mayonnaise
- 1 teaspoon of lemon juice
- 4 large lettuce leaves

Cooking Instructions:

1. In a bowl, combine tuna, celery, red bell peppers, mayonnaise, and lemon juice.
2. Mix until well combined.
3. Spoon the tuna salad into lettuce leaves, creating wraps.

Nutritional Information (per serving):

- Calories: 120
- Protein: 15g
- Carbohydrates: 3g
- Fiber: 1g
- Potassium: 220mg

TURKEY AND AVOCADO WRAP

Benefit: High in protein and healthy fats, low in sodium.

- Prep/Cook Time: 15 minutes
- Servings: 2

Ingredients:

- 4 ounces of low-sodium turkey breast slices
- 1 small avocado, sliced
- 1/2 cup of baby spinach
- 2 whole-wheat tortillas (low sodium)

Cooking Instructions:

1. Lay out the tortillas and layer each with turkey slices, avocado, and baby spinach.
2. Roll up the tortillas, securing them with toothpicks if needed.
3. Slice in half and serve.

Nutritional Information (per serving):

- Calories: 300
- Protein: 20g
- Carbohydrates: 20g
- Fiber: 6g
- Potassium: 450mg

LEMON HERB BAKED SALMON

Benefit: High in omega-3 fatty acids, low in sodium and potassium.

- Prep/Cook Time: 25 minutes
- Servings: 2

Ingredients:

- 2 salmon fillets (4 ounces each)
- 1 lemon, sliced
- 2 cloves of garlic, minced
- 1 teaspoon of dried dill
- Salt and pepper to taste

Cooking Instructions:

1. Preheat the oven to 375°F (190°C).
2. Place salmon fillets on a baking sheet lined with foil.
3. Season with minced garlic, dried dill, salt, and pepper.
4. Top with lemon slices.
5. Bake for 15-20 minutes until salmon flakes easily with a fork.

Nutritional Information (per serving):

- Calories: 250
- Protein: 25g
- Carbohydrates: 3g
- Fiber: 1g
- Potassium: 350mg

MEDITERRANEAN CHICKPEA SALAD

Benefit: High in fiber, low in sodium and potassium.

- Prep/Cook Time: 15 minutes
- Servings: 4

Ingredients:

- 2 cans (15 ounces each) of low-sodium chickpeas, drained and rinsed
- 1 cup of diced cucumbers
- 1 cup of diced tomatoes
- 1/2 cup of diced red onions
- 1/4 cup of chopped fresh parsley
- 2 tablespoons of olive oil
- 2 tablespoons of lemon juice
- Salt and pepper to taste

Cooking Instructions:

1. In a large bowl, combine chickpeas, cucumbers, tomatoes, red onions, and parsley.
2. Drizzle with olive oil and lemon juice.
3. Season with salt and pepper, and toss to coat.
4. Serve chilled.

Nutritional Information (per serving):

- Calories: 280
- Protein: 11g
- Carbohydrates: 42g
- Fiber: 11g
- Potassium: 490mg

VEGETABLE AND BROWN RICE STIR-FRY

Benefit: High in fiber, customizable with kidney-friendly vegetables.

- Prep/Cook Time: 30 minutes
- Servings: 4

Ingredients:

- 1 cup of cooked brown rice
- 2 cups of mixed kidney-friendly vegetables (e.g., broccoli, bell peppers, snap peas)
- 1/4 cup of low-sodium soy sauce
- 1 tablespoon of olive oil
- 2 cloves of garlic, minced
- 1 teaspoon of ginger, minced

Cooking Instructions:

1. In a wok or large skillet, heat olive oil over medium-high heat.
2. Add minced garlic and ginger, and sauté for a minute.
3. Add the mixed vegetables and stir-fry until tender-crisp.
4. Stir in cooked brown rice and soy sauce, and cook until heated through.
5. Serve hot.

Nutritional Information (per serving):

- Calories: 200
- Protein: 5g
- Carbohydrates: 35g
- Fiber: 4g
- Potassium: 250mg

LENTIL AND SPINACH SOUP

Benefit: High in protein, low in sodium and potassium.

- Prep/Cook Time: 45 minutes
- Servings: 4

Ingredients:

- 1 cup of dry green lentils, rinsed and drained
- 4 cups of low-sodium vegetable broth
- 2 cups of chopped fresh spinach
- 1/2 cup of diced carrots
- 1/2 cup of diced celery
- 1/2 cup of diced onions
- 2 cloves of garlic, minced
- 1 teaspoon of cumin
- Salt and pepper to taste

Cooking Instructions:

1. In a large pot, sauté onions, carrots, celery, and garlic until softened.
2. Add lentils, vegetable broth, cumin, salt, and pepper.
3. Simmer for 30-35 minutes until lentils are tender.
4. Stir in chopped spinach and cook until wilted.
5. Serve hot.

Nutritional Information (per serving):

- Calories: 220
- Protein: 15g
- Carbohydrates: 38g
- Fiber: 14g
- Potassium: 570mg

TOFU AND VEGETABLE STIR-FRY

Benefit: High in protein, customizable with kidney-friendly vegetables.

- Prep/Cook Time: 30 minutes
- Servings: 4

Ingredients:

- 1 block (14 ounces) of firm tofu, cubed
- 2 cups of mixed kidney-friendly vegetables (e.g., snow peas, carrots, bell peppers)
- 1/4 cup of low-sodium stir-fry sauce
- 2 tablespoons of vegetable oil
- 2 cloves of garlic, minced
- Cooked brown rice for serving

Cooking Instructions:

1. Heat vegetable oil in a wok or large skillet over medium-high heat.
2. Add minced garlic and cubed tofu, stir-fry until tofu is lightly browned.
3. Add mixed vegetables and stir-fry until tender-crisp.
4. Pour in stir-fry sauce and cook until heated through.
5. Serve over cooked brown rice.

Nutritional Information (per serving):

- Calories: 250
- Protein: 14g
- Carbohydrates: 20g
- Fiber: 4g
- Potassium: 450mg

LEMON DILL SHRIMP SKEWERS

Benefit: High in protein, low in sodium and potassium.

- Prep/Cook Time: 20 minutes
- Servings: 2

Ingredients:

- 1/2 pound of large shrimp, peeled and deveined
- Zest and juice of 1 lemon
- 1 tablespoon of olive oil
- 1 teaspoon of dried dill
- Salt and pepper to taste
- Wooden skewers, soaked in water

Cooking Instructions:

1. In a bowl, whisk together lemon zest, lemon juice, olive oil, dried dill, salt, and pepper.
2. Thread shrimp onto wooden skewers.
3. Brush the shrimp with the lemon dill mixture.
4. Grill the shrimp skewers for 2-3 minutes per side or until they turn pink and opaque.
5. Serve hot.

Nutritional Information (per serving):

- Calories: 160
- Protein: 20g
- Carbohydrates: 2g
- Fiber: 0g
- Potassium: 200mg

DINNER RECIPES

STUFFED BELL PEPPERS

Benefit: High in fiber, low in sodium and potassium.

- Prep/Cook Time: 1 hour
- Servings: 4

Ingredients:

- 4 large bell peppers
- 1 cup of cooked brown rice
- 1/2 cup of cooked lean ground turkey
- 1/2 cup of low-sodium tomato sauce
- 1/4 cup of diced onions
- 1/4 cup of diced zucchini
- 1/4 cup of diced carrots
- Salt and pepper to taste

Cooking Instructions:

1. Preheat the oven to 350°F (175°C).
2. Cut the tops off the bell peppers and remove seeds.
3. In a bowl, combine cooked brown rice, ground turkey, diced vegetables, and tomato sauce.
4. Season with salt and pepper.
5. Stuff each bell pepper with the mixture.
6. Place stuffed peppers in a baking dish, cover with foil, and bake for 40-45 minutes until peppers are tender.

Nutritional Information (per serving):

- Calories: 220
- Protein: 15g
- Carbohydrates: 35g
- Fiber: 6g

- Potassium: 390mg

LEMON GARLIC SHRIMP AND ASPARAGUS

Benefit: High in protein, low in sodium and potassium.

- Prep/Cook Time: 30 minutes
- Servings: 2

Ingredients:

- 1/2 pound of large shrimp, peeled and deveined
- 1 bunch of asparagus, trimmed
- Zest and juice of 1 lemon
- 2 cloves of garlic, minced
- 1 tablespoon of olive oil
- Salt and pepper to taste

Cooking Instructions:

1. In a bowl, whisk together lemon zest, lemon juice, minced garlic, olive oil, salt, and pepper.
2. Toss shrimp and asparagus with the lemon garlic mixture.
3. Heat a skillet over medium-high heat.
4. Cook shrimp and asparagus for 2-3 minutes per side until shrimp are pink and opaque.
5. Serve hot.

Nutritional Information (per serving):

- Calories: 220
- Protein: 25g
- Carbohydrates: 10g
- Fiber: 4g
- Potassium: 340mg

CAULIFLOWER AND SPINACH CURRY

Benefit: Low in potassium, high in fiber and antioxidants.

- Prep/Cook Time: 40 minutes
- Servings: 4

Ingredients:

- 1 medium cauliflower, cut into florets
- 4 cups of fresh spinach leaves
- 1 can (14 ounces) of low-sodium diced tomatoes
- 1 can (14 ounces) of chickpeas, drained and rinsed
- 1 onion, finely chopped
- 2 cloves of garlic, minced
- 1 tablespoon of olive oil
- 2 tablespoons of curry powder
- Salt and pepper to taste

Cooking Instructions:

1. In a large skillet, heat olive oil over medium heat.
2. Add chopped onions and minced garlic, and sauté until onions are translucent.
3. Stir in curry powder and cook for another minute.
4. Add cauliflower florets, diced tomatoes, and chickpeas. Simmer for 15-20 minutes until cauliflower is tender.
5. Add fresh spinach and cook until wilted.
6. Season with salt and pepper.
7. Serve hot over cooked brown rice.

Nutritional Information (per serving):

- Calories: 230
- Protein: 10g
- Carbohydrates: 40g
- Fiber: 11g
- Potassium: 570mg

MUSHROOM AND QUINOA STUFFED ACORN SQUASH

Benefit: High in fiber and antioxidants, low in sodium and potassium.

- Prep/Cook Time: 1 hour
- Servings: 2

Ingredients:

- 1 acorn squash, halved and seeds removed
- 1 cup of cooked quinoa
- 1 cup of sliced mushrooms
- 1/4 cup of diced onions
- 2 cloves of garlic, minced
- 2 tablespoons of grated Parmesan cheese (optional)
- 1 tablespoon of olive oil
- Salt and pepper to taste

Cooking Instructions:

1. Preheat the oven to 375°F (190°C).
2. Brush the cut sides of the acorn squash with olive oil and sprinkle with salt and pepper.
3. Place squash halves on a baking sheet, cut side down, and bake for 30-35 minutes until tender.
4. In a skillet, sauté onions, garlic, and mushrooms until mushrooms are browned.
5. Stir in cooked quinoa and heat through.
6. Fill the roasted acorn squash halves with the quinoa and mushroom mixture.
7. Sprinkle with grated Parmesan cheese if desired.
8. Return to the oven for 10 minutes to melt the cheese.
9. Serve hot.

Nutritional Information (per serving):

- Calories: 350
- Protein: 10g
- Carbohydrates: 60g
- Fiber: 10g
- Potassium: 790mg

LEMON HERB BAKED COD

Benefit: High in protein, low in sodium and potassium.

- Prep/Cook Time: 25 minutes
- Servings: 2

Ingredients:

- 2 cod fillets (4 ounces each)
- Zest and juice of 1 lemon
- 2 cloves of garlic, minced
- 1 teaspoon of dried thyme
- 1 tablespoon of olive oil
- Salt and pepper to taste

Cooking Instructions:

1. Preheat the oven to 375°F (190°C).
2. In a bowl, whisk together lemon zest, lemon juice, minced garlic, dried thyme, olive oil, salt, and pepper.
3. Place cod fillets on a baking sheet lined with foil.
4. Pour the lemon herb mixture over the cod.
5. Bake for 15-20 minutes until the cod flakes easily with a fork.
6. Serve hot.

Nutritional Information (per serving):

- Calories: 160
- Protein: 25g
- Carbohydrates: 3g
- Fiber: 1g
- Potassium: 350mg

SPAGHETTI SQUASH PRIMAVERA

Benefit: Low in potassium, high in fiber and vitamins.

- Prep/Cook Time: 45 minutes
- Servings: 4

Ingredients:

- 1 spaghetti squash, halved and seeds removed
- 2 cups of mixed kidney-friendly vegetables (e.g., bell peppers, broccoli, carrots)
- 2 cloves of garlic, minced
- 1/4 cup of low-sodium vegetable broth
- 2 tablespoons of olive oil
- 1/4 cup of grated Parmesan cheese (optional)
- Salt and pepper to taste

Cooking Instructions:

1. Preheat the oven to 375°F (190°C).
2. Brush the cut sides of the spaghetti squash with olive oil and sprinkle with salt and pepper.
3. Place squash halves on a baking sheet, cut side down, and bake for 30-35 minutes until tender.
4. In a skillet, sauté minced garlic and mixed vegetables until they are tender-crisp.
5. Scrape the cooked spaghetti squash flesh into strands with a fork.
6. Toss the spaghetti squash with sautéed vegetables and vegetable broth.
7. Sprinkle with grated Parmesan cheese if desired.
8. Serve hot.

Nutritional Information (per serving):

- Calories: 180
- Protein: 4g
- Carbohydrates: 20g
- Fiber: 5g
- Potassium: 320mg

LENTIL AND SWEET POTATO CURRY

Benefit: High in fiber and plant-based protein, low in sodium and potassium.

- Prep/Cook Time: 45 minutes
- Servings: 4

Ingredients:

- 1 cup of dry green or brown lentils, rinsed and drained
- 2 sweet potatoes, peeled and diced
- 1 can (14 ounces) of low-sodium diced tomatoes
- 1 can (14 ounces) of light coconut milk
- 1 onion, finely chopped
- 2 cloves of garlic, minced
- 2 tablespoons of curry powder
- 1 tablespoon of olive oil
- Salt and pepper to taste

Cooking Instructions:

1. In a large pot, heat olive oil over medium heat.
2. Add chopped onions and minced garlic, and sauté until onions are translucent.
3. Stir in curry powder and cook for another minute.
4. Add diced sweet potatoes, lentils, diced tomatoes, and coconut milk.
5. Simmer for 25-30 minutes until sweet potatoes are tender and lentils are cooked.
6. Season with salt and pepper.
7. Serve hot over cooked brown rice.

Nutritional Information (per serving):

- Calories: 350
- Protein: 15g
- Carbohydrates: 60g
- Fiber: 12g
- Potassium: 760mg

BAKED EGGPLANT PARMESAN

Benefit: Low in sodium and potassium, a kidney-friendly twist on a classic Italian dish.

- Prep/Cook Time: 1 hour
- Servings: 4

Ingredients:

- 1 large eggplant, sliced into rounds
- 1 cup of low-sodium marinara sauce
- 1 cup of shredded mozzarella cheese (low sodium)
- 1/4 cup of grated Parmesan cheese
- 1/4 cup of whole-wheat bread crumbs
- 1/4 cup of fresh basil leaves
- 1 egg, beaten
- Olive oil cooking spray
- Salt and pepper to taste

Cooking Instructions:

1. Preheat the oven to 375°F (190°C).
2. Place eggplant slices on a baking sheet, sprinkle with salt, and let sit for 10 minutes.
3. Rinse the eggplant slices and pat dry with a paper towel.
4. In a shallow dish, mix together bread crumbs, grated Parmesan cheese, and fresh basil.
5. Dip each eggplant slice into the beaten egg, then coat with the breadcrumb mixture.
6. Lay the breaded eggplant slices on a baking sheet coated with olive oil cooking spray.
7. Bake for 25-30 minutes until the eggplant is tender and golden.
8. In a baking dish, layer marinara sauce, baked eggplant slices, and shredded mozzarella cheese.
9. Repeat the layers.
10. Bake for an additional 20 minutes until the cheese is bubbly and golden.
11. Serve hot.

Nutritional Information (per serving):

- Calories: 300
- Protein: 15g
- Carbohydrates: 30g
- Fiber: 8g
- Potassium: 450mg

GRILLED PORTOBELLO MUSHROOMS WITH BALSAMIC GLAZE

Benefit: Low in sodium and potassium, a flavorful and hearty vegetarian option.

- Prep/Cook Time: 30 minutes
- Servings: 2

Ingredients:

- 2 large portobello mushrooms, cleaned and stems removed
- 1/4 cup of balsamic vinegar (low sodium)
- 2 cloves of garlic, minced
- 2 tablespoons of olive oil
- 1 teaspoon of dried thyme
- Salt and pepper to taste

Cooking Instructions:

1. In a bowl, whisk together balsamic vinegar, minced garlic, olive oil, dried thyme, salt, and pepper.
2. Brush the portobello mushrooms with the balsamic mixture.
3. Preheat the grill to medium-high heat.
4. Grill the mushrooms for 4-5 minutes per side until tender.
5. Serve hot.

Nutritional Information (per serving):

- Calories: 160
- Protein: 4g
- Carbohydrates: 10g
- Fiber: 2g
- Potassium: 320mg

QUINOA AND BLACK BEAN STUFFED PEPPERS

Benefit: High in fiber and plant-based protein, low in sodium and potassium.

- Prep/Cook Time: 1 hour
- Servings: 4

Ingredients

- 4 large bell peppers
- 1 cup of cooked quinoa
- 1 can (15 ounces) of low-sodium black beans, drained and rinsed
- 1 cup of diced tomatoes
- 1/2 cup of diced red onions
- 1/2 cup of corn kernels (fresh or frozen)
- 1/4 cup of chopped fresh cilantro
- 1 teaspoon of ground cumin
- Salt and pepper to taste

Cooking Instructions:

1. Cut the tops off the bell peppers and remove seeds.
2. In a bowl, combine cooked quinoa, black beans, diced tomatoes, diced red onions, corn kernels, chopped cilantro, ground cumin, salt, and pepper.
3. Stuff each bell pepper with the quinoa and black bean mixture.
4. Place stuffed peppers in a baking dish, cover with foil, and bake for 40-45 minutes until peppers are tender.
5. Serve hot.

Nutritional Information (per serving):

- Calories: 320
- Protein: 12g
- Carbohydrates: 60g
- Fiber: 12g
- Potassium: 540mg

SNACKS AND APPETIZERS

HUMMUS AND VEGGIE PLATTER

Benefit: Low in sodium and potassium, high in fiber and protein.

- Prep Time: 10 minutes
- Servings: 4

Ingredients:

- 1 cup of low-sodium hummus
- Assorted fresh vegetables (carrot sticks, cucumber slices, bell pepper strips)

Cooking Instructions:

1. Arrange the fresh vegetables on a platter.
2. Serve with a bowl of low-sodium hummus for dipping.

Nutritional Information (per serving):

- Calories: 150
- Protein: 6g
- Carbohydrates: 18g
- Fiber: 6g
- Potassium: 300mg

CUCUMBER AND GREEK YOGURT DIP

Benefit: Low in sodium and potassium, high in protein.

- Prep Time: 10 minutes
- Servings: 4

Ingredients:

- 1 cucumber, peeled and diced
- 1 cup of low-fat Greek yogurt
- 1 clove of garlic, minced

- 1 tablespoon of fresh dill, chopped
- Salt and pepper to taste

Cooking Instructions:

1. In a bowl, combine diced cucumber, Greek yogurt, minced garlic, and chopped dill.
2. Season with salt and pepper.
3. Chill in the refrigerator before serving.

Nutritional Information (per serving):

- Calories: 70
- Protein: 7g
- Carbohydrates: 8g
- Fiber: 1g
- Potassium: 180mg

STUFFED CELERY STICKS

Benefit: Low in sodium and potassium, a crunchy and satisfying snack.

- Prep Time: 15 minutes
- Servings: 4

Ingredients:

- 4 celery stalks, cut into sticks
- 1/2 cup of low-fat cream cheese
- 2 tablespoons of chopped chives
- 2 tablespoons of chopped walnuts (optional)

Cooking Instructions:

1. In a bowl, mix low-fat cream cheese and chopped chives.
2. Fill celery sticks with the cream cheese mixture.
3. Optionally, sprinkle with chopped walnuts.

Nutritional Information (per serving):

- Calories: 90
- Protein: 4g
- Carbohydrates: 3g
- Fiber: 1g
- Potassium: 160mg

BAKED SWEET POTATO FRIES

Benefit: Low in sodium and potassium, a tasty alternative to regular fries.

- Prep/Cook Time: 30 minutes
- Servings: 4

Ingredients:

- 2 sweet potatoes, cut into fries
- 1 tablespoon of olive oil
- 1 teaspoon of paprika
- Salt and pepper to taste

Cooking Instructions:

1. Preheat the oven to 425°F (220°C).
2. Toss sweet potato fries with olive oil, paprika, salt, and pepper.
3. Spread them in a single layer on a baking sheet.
4. Bake for 20-25 minutes until crispy, flipping once.

Nutritional Information (per serving):

- Calories: 100
- Protein: 2g
- Carbohydrates: 19g
- Fiber: 3g
- Potassium: 270mg

ROASTED CHICKPEAS

Benefit: High in protein and fiber, low in sodium and potassium.

- Prep/Cook Time: 40 minutes
- Servings: 4

Ingredients:

- 1 can (15 ounces) of low-sodium chickpeas, drained and rinsed
- 1 tablespoon of olive oil
- 1 teaspoon of paprika
- 1/2 teaspoon of cumin
- 1/2 teaspoon of garlic powder
- Salt and pepper to taste

Cooking Instructions:

- Preheat the oven to 400°F (200°C).
- Pat chickpeas dry with a paper towel.
- Toss chickpeas with olive oil, paprika, cumin, garlic powder, salt, and pepper.
- Spread them on a baking sheet.
- Roast for 30-35 minutes until crispy, shaking the pan occasionally.

Nutritional Information (per serving):

- Calories: 120
- Protein: 5g
- Carbohydrates: 15g
- Fiber: 4g
- Potassium: 180mg

MOZZARELLA AND TOMATO SKEWERS

Benefit: Low in sodium and potassium, a simple and flavorful appetizer.

- Prep Time: 10 minutes
- Servings: 4

Ingredients:

- 8 cherry tomatoes
- 8 small fresh mozzarella balls
- Fresh basil leaves
- Balsamic vinegar glaze (low sodium)

Cooking Instructions:

1. Thread a cherry tomato, a fresh mozzarella ball, and a basil leaf onto a skewer.
2. Drizzle with balsamic vinegar glaze.
3. Repeat for all skewers.

Nutritional Information (per serving):

- Calories: 90
- Protein: 6g
- Carbohydrates: 2g
- Fiber: 1g
- Potassium: 100mg

AVOCADO AND TOMATO SALSA

Benefit: Low in sodium and potassium, a creamy and refreshing dip.

- Prep Time: 15 minutes
- Servings: 4

Ingredients:

- 2 ripe avocados, diced
- 2 tomatoes, diced

- 1/4 cup of diced red onions
- 2 tablespoons of fresh cilantro, chopped
- 1 lime, juiced
- Salt and pepper to taste

Cooking Instructions:

1. In a bowl, gently combine diced avocados, diced tomatoes, diced red onions, and chopped cilantro.
2. Drizzle with lime juice and season with salt and pepper.
3. Serve with tortilla chips or whole-grain crackers.

Nutritional Information (per serving):

- Calories: 120
- Protein: 2g
- Carbohydrates: 7g
- Fiber: 5g
- Potassium: 330mg

SPINACH AND ARTICHOKE DIP (LOW SODIUM VERSION)

Benefit: A kidney-friendly twist on a classic favorite, lower in sodium.

- Prep/Cook Time: 25 minutes
- Servings: 4

Ingredients:

- 1 cup of chopped frozen spinach, thawed and drained
- 1 can (14 ounces) of artichoke hearts, drained and chopped
- 1 cup of low-fat sour cream
- 1/2 cup of grated Parmesan cheese (low sodium)
- 1/4 cup of mayonnaise
- 1 clove of garlic, minced
- Salt and pepper to taste

Cooking Instructions:

1. Preheat the oven to 350°F (175°C).
2. In a bowl, mix chopped spinach, chopped artichoke hearts, low-fat sour cream, grated Parmesan cheese, mayonnaise, minced garlic, salt, and pepper.
3. Transfer the mixture to a baking dish.
4. Bake for 20 minutes or until bubbly and lightly browned.
5. Serve with whole-grain crackers or fresh vegetable sticks.

Nutritional Information (per serving):

- Calories: 220
- Protein: 10g
- Carbohydrates: 12g
- Fiber: 3g
- Potassium: 240mg

BAKED ZUCCHINI CHIPS

Benefit: Low in sodium and potassium, a crispy and satisfying snack.

- Prep/Cook Time: 30 minutes
- Servings: 4

Ingredients:

- 2 large zucchinis, thinly sliced
- 2 tablespoons of olive oil
- 1/4 cup of grated Parmesan cheese (low sodium)
- 1/4 cup of whole-wheat bread crumbs
- 1/2 teaspoon of garlic powder
- Salt and pepper to taste

Cooking Instructions:

1. Preheat the oven to 425°F (220°C).

2. In a bowl, toss zucchini slices with olive oil, grated Parmesan cheese, whole-wheat bread crumbs, garlic powder, salt, and pepper.
3. Place zucchini slices on a baking sheet in a single layer.
4. Bake for 20-25 minutes until golden and crispy.

Nutritional Information (per serving):

- Calories: 130
- Protein: 5g
- Carbohydrates: 9g
- Fiber: 2g
- Potassium: 370mg

SLICED APPLE WITH ALMOND BUTTER

Benefit: A simple, no-cook option, low in sodium and potassium.

- Prep Time: 5 minutes
- Servings: 2

Ingredients:

- 1 apple, sliced
- 2 tablespoons of almond butter (unsalted)

Cooking Instructions:

1. Slice the apple into thin wedges.
2. Serve with almond butter for dipping or spreading.

Nutritional Information (per serving):

- Calories: 180
- Protein: 4g
- Carbohydrates: 20g
- Fiber: 4g
- Potassium: 200mg

MAIN COURSES (INCLUDING VEGETARIAN OPTIONS)

GRILLED LEMON HERB CHICKEN

Benefit: High in protein, low in sodium and potassium.

- Prep/Cook Time: 30 minutes
- Servings: 4

Ingredients:

- 4 boneless, skinless chicken breasts (4 ounces each)
- Zest and juice of 1 lemon
- 2 cloves of garlic, minced
- 1 teaspoon of dried thyme
- 1 teaspoon of dried rosemary
- 1 tablespoon of olive oil
- Salt and pepper to taste

Cooking Instructions:

1. In a bowl, whisk together lemon zest, lemon juice, minced garlic, dried thyme, dried rosemary, olive oil, salt, and pepper.
2. Coat chicken breasts with the lemon herb mixture.
3. Preheat the grill to medium-high heat.
4. Grill chicken for 6-8 minutes per side until cooked through.
5. Serve hot.

Nutritional Information (per serving):

- Calories: 180
- Protein: 25g
- Carbohydrates: 1g
- Fiber: 0g
- Potassium: 240mg

EGGPLANT PARMESAN (VEGETARIAN)

Benefit: A kidney-friendly twist on a classic Italian dish, low in sodium and potassium.

- Prep/Cook Time: 1 hour
- Servings: 4

Ingredients:

- 1 large eggplant, sliced into rounds
- 1 cup of low-sodium marinara sauce
- 1 cup of shredded mozzarella cheese (low sodium)
- 1/4 cup of grated Parmesan cheese
- 1/4 cup of whole-wheat bread crumbs
- 1/4 cup of fresh basil leaves
- 1 egg, beaten
- Olive oil cooking spray
- Salt and pepper to taste

Cooking Instructions:

1. Preheat the oven to 375°F (190°C).
2. Place eggplant slices on a baking sheet, sprinkle with salt, and let sit for 10 minutes.
3. Rinse the eggplant slices and pat dry with a paper towel.
4. In a shallow dish, mix together bread crumbs, grated Parmesan cheese, and fresh basil.
5. Dip each eggplant slice into the beaten egg, then coat with the breadcrumb mixture.
6. Lay the breaded eggplant slices on a baking sheet coated with olive oil cooking spray.
7. Bake for 25-30 minutes until the eggplant is tender and golden.
8. In a baking dish, layer marinara sauce, baked eggplant slices, and shredded mozzarella cheese.
9. Repeat the layers.
10. Bake for an additional 20 minutes until the cheese is bubbly and golden. Serve hot.

Nutritional Information (per serving):

- Calories: 300

- Protein: 15g
- Carbohydrates: 30g
- Fiber: 8g
- Potassium: 450mg

LENTIL AND VEGETABLE STIR-FRY (VEGETARIAN)

Benefit: High in protein and fiber, low in sodium and potassium.

- Prep/Cook Time: 30 minutes
- Servings: 4

Ingredients:

- 1 cup of dry green or brown lentils, rinsed and drained
- 2 cups of mixed kidney-friendly vegetables (e.g., bell peppers, broccoli, carrots)
- 2 cloves of garlic, minced
- 1/4 cup of low-sodium vegetable broth
- 2 tablespoons of low-sodium soy sauce
- 1 tablespoon of olive oil
- 1/2 teaspoon of ground ginger
- Salt and pepper to taste

Cooking Instructions:

1. In a saucepan, cook lentils according to package instructions.
2. In a large skillet, heat olive oil over medium-high heat.
3. Add minced garlic and sauté for 1 minute.
4. Add mixed vegetables and sauté until they are tender-crisp.
5. Stir in cooked lentils, low-sodium vegetable broth, low-sodium soy sauce, ground ginger, salt, and pepper.
6. Cook for 5-7 minutes until heated through.
7. Serve hot over cooked brown rice.

Nutritional Information (per serving):

- Calories: 320
- Protein: 15g
- Carbohydrates: 60g
- Fiber: 12g
- Potassium: 540mg

BAKED SALMON WITH DILL SAUCE

Benefit: High in omega-3 fatty acids and protein, low in sodium and potassium.

- Prep/Cook Time: 25 minutes
- Servings: 4

Ingredients:

- 4 salmon fillets (4 ounces each)
- Zest and juice of 1 lemon
- 2 tablespoons of fresh dill, chopped
- 1/4 cup of low-fat sour cream
- 1 clove of garlic, minced
- Salt and pepper to taste

Cooking Instructions:

1. Preheat the oven to 375°F (190°C).
2. Place salmon fillets on a baking sheet.
3. In a bowl, whisk together lemon zest, lemon juice, chopped dill, low-fat sour cream, minced garlic, salt, and pepper.
4. Spread the dill sauce over the salmon fillets.
5. Bake for 15-18 minutes until salmon flakes easily with a fork.
6. Serve hot.

Nutritional Information (per serving):

- Calories: 220
- Protein: 25g

- Carbohydrates: 3g
- Fiber: 0g
- Potassium: 380mg

SPINACH AND MUSHROOM RISOTTO (VEGETARIAN)

Benefit: Creamy and comforting, low in sodium and potassium.

- Prep/Cook Time: 45 minutes
- Servings: 4

Ingredients:

- 1 cup of Arborio rice
- 1/2 cup of dry white wine (optional)
- 4 cups of low-sodium vegetable broth
- 2 cups of fresh spinach, chopped
- 1 cup of mushrooms, sliced
- 1/2 cup of diced onions
- 2 cloves of garlic, minced
- 2 tablespoons of olive oil
- 1/4 cup of grated Parmesan cheese (low sodium)
- Salt and pepper to taste

Cooking Instructions:

1. In a saucepan, heat low-sodium vegetable broth and keep it warm over low heat.
2. In a large skillet, heat olive oil over medium heat.
3. Add diced onions and sliced mushrooms, and sauté until they are soft.
4. Stir in Arborio rice and minced garlic, and cook for 2 minutes.
5. If using, pour in the dry white wine and cook until it is absorbed by the rice.
6. Begin adding the warm vegetable broth, one ladle at a time, stirring frequently and allowing the liquid to be absorbed before adding more.
7. Continue this process until the rice is tender and creamy (about 20-25 minutes).
8. Stir in chopped spinach and grated Parmesan cheese until spinach wilts.

9. Season with salt and pepper.
10. Serve hot.

Nutritional Information (per serving):

- Calories: 290
- Protein: 8g
- Carbohydrates: 44g
- Fiber: 2g
- Potassium: 270mg

TURKEY AND VEGETABLE STIR-FRY

Benefit: High in protein, low in sodium and potassium.

- Prep/Cook Time: 25 minutes
- Servings: 4

Ingredients:

- 1 pound of ground turkey
- 2 cups of mixed kidney-friendly vegetables (e.g., bell peppers, broccoli, carrots)
- 1/4 cup of low-sodium teriyaki sauce
- 1 tablespoon of olive oil
- 2 cloves of garlic, minced
- Salt and pepper to taste

Cooking Instructions:

1. In a large skillet, heat olive oil over medium-high heat.
2. Add minced garlic and sauté for 1 minute.
3. Add ground turkey and cook until browned, breaking it into crumbles.
4. Stir in mixed vegetables and low-sodium teriyaki sauce.
5. Cook for 5-7 minutes until vegetables are tender.
6. Season with salt and pepper.
7. Serve hot over cooked brown rice.

Nutritional Information (per serving):

- Calories: 250
- Protein: 28g
- Carbohydrates: 10g
- Fiber: 3g
- Potassium: 320mg

SWEET POTATO AND BLACK BEAN TACOS (VEGETARIAN)

Benefit: High in fiber and plant-based protein, low in sodium and potassium.

- Prep/Cook Time: 30 minutes
- Servings: 4

Ingredients:

- 2 large sweet potatoes, peeled and diced
- 1 can (15 ounces) of low-sodium black beans, drained and rinsed
- 1 cup of diced tomatoes
- 1/2 cup of diced red onions
- 2 teaspoons of ground cumin
- 1 teaspoon of chili powder
- 1/4 cup of fresh cilantro, chopped
- 8 small whole-wheat tortillas
- Olive oil cooking spray
- Salt and pepper to taste

Cooking Instructions:

1. Preheat the oven to 425°F (220°C).
2. Toss diced sweet potatoes with olive oil, ground cumin, chili powder, salt, and pepper.
3. Spread sweet potatoes on a baking sheet and roast for 20-25 minutes until tender and slightly crispy.
4. In a bowl, combine black beans, diced tomatoes, diced red onions, and chopped cilantro.
5. Warm whole-wheat tortillas in a skillet or microwave.
6. Assemble tacos by filling each tortilla with roasted sweet potatoes and the black bean mixture.

7. Serve hot.

Nutritional Information (per serving):

- Calories: 330
- Protein: 10g
- Carbohydrates: 60g
- Fiber: 12g
- Potassium: 530mg

LEMON GARLIC ROASTED TOFU AND VEGETABLES (VEGAN)

Benefit: High in plant-based protein, low in sodium and potassium.

- Prep/Cook Time: 40 minutes
- Servings: 4

Ingredients:

- 1 block (14 ounces) of extra-firm tofu, cubed
- 4 cups of mixed kidney-friendly vegetables (e.g., bell peppers, broccoli, and carrots)
- Zest and juice of 1 lemon
- 2 cloves of garlic, minced
- 2 tablespoons of olive oil
- Salt and pepper to taste

Cooking Instructions:

1. Preheat the oven to 425°F (220°C).
2. In a bowl, whisk together lemon zest, lemon juice, minced garlic, olive oil, salt, and pepper.
3. Toss tofu cubes and mixed vegetables with the lemon garlic mixture.
4. Spread them on a baking sheet.
5. Roast for 25-30 minutes until tofu is crispy and vegetables are tender. Serve hot.

Nutritional Information (per serving):

Calories: 240 | Protein: 15g | Carbohydrates: 20g | Fiber: 5g | Potassium: 450mg

SOUPS AND SALADS RECIPES

CREAMY CAULIFLOWER SOUP

Benefit: Low in sodium and potassium, a creamy and satisfying soup.

- Prep/Cook Time: 45 minutes
- Servings: 4

Ingredients:

- 1 head of cauliflower, chopped
- 1 small onion, chopped
- 2 cloves of garlic, minced
- 4 cups of low-sodium vegetable broth
- 1 cup of low-fat milk
- 2 tablespoons of olive oil
- Salt and pepper to taste

Cooking Instructions:

1. In a large pot, heat olive oil over medium heat.
2. Add chopped onion and minced garlic, sauté until softened.
3. Add cauliflower and low-sodium vegetable broth.
4. Simmer for 20-25 minutes until cauliflower is tender.
5. Use an immersion blender to blend until smooth.
6. Stir in low-fat milk and heat until warmed through.
7. Season with salt and pepper.
8. Serve hot.

Nutritional Information (per serving):

- Calories: 110
- Protein: 4g
- Carbohydrates: 15g
- Fiber: 5g
- Potassium: 470mg

ROASTED RED PEPPER AND LENTIL SOUP

Benefit: High in protein and fiber, low in sodium and potassium.

- Prep/Cook Time: 1 hour
- Servings: 4

Ingredients:

- 2 red bell peppers
- 1 cup of dry red lentils, rinsed and drained
- 1 small onion, chopped
- 2 cloves of garlic, minced
- 4 cups of low-sodium vegetable broth
- 1 teaspoon of cumin
- 1/2 teaspoon of smoked paprika
- 2 tablespoons of olive oil
- Salt and pepper to taste

Cooking Instructions:

1. Preheat the oven to 425°F (220°C).
2. Place red bell peppers on a baking sheet and roast for 25-30 minutes until skin is charred.
3. Remove peppers from the oven, place them in a covered bowl to steam, and then peel and chop them.
4. In a large pot, heat olive oil over medium heat.
5. Add chopped onion and minced garlic, sauté until softened.
6. Stir in roasted red peppers, red lentils, low-sodium vegetable broth, cumin, and smoked paprika.
7. Simmer for 25-30 minutes until lentils are tender.
8. Use an immersion blender to blend until smooth.
9. Season with salt and pepper.
10. Serve hot.

Nutritional Information (per serving):

- Calories: 270
- Protein: 13g
- Carbohydrates: 40g
- Fiber: 10g
- Potassium: 440mg

GREEK QUINOA SALAD

Benefit: High in protein and fiber, low in sodium and potassium.

- Prep Time: 15 minutes
- Servings: 4

Ingredients:

- 1 cup of cooked quinoa
- 1 cup of cucumber, diced
- 1 cup of cherry tomatoes, halved
- 1/2 cup of diced red onions
- 1/4 cup of chopped fresh parsley
- 1/4 cup of crumbled feta cheese (low sodium)
- 2 tablespoons of extra-virgin olive oil
- Juice of 1 lemon
- 1 teaspoon of dried oregano
- Salt and pepper to taste

Cooking Instructions:

1. In a large bowl, combine cooked quinoa, diced cucumber, cherry tomatoes, diced red onions, chopped parsley, and crumbled feta cheese.
2. Drizzle with extra-virgin olive oil and lemon juice.
3. Sprinkle dried oregano over the salad.
4. Season with salt and pepper.
5. Toss to combine.
6. Serve cold.

Nutritional Information (per serving):

- Calories: 260
- Protein: 7g
- Carbohydrates: 30g
- Fiber: 4g
- Potassium: 320mg

CHICKEN AND RICE SOUP

Benefit: Comforting and low in sodium and potassium.

- Prep/Cook Time: 40 minutes
- Servings: 4

Ingredients:

- 1 pound of boneless, skinless chicken thighs
- 1 cup of white rice
- 4 cups of low-sodium chicken broth
- 1 cup of carrots, sliced
- 1 cup of celery, sliced
- 1 small onion, chopped
- 2 cloves of garlic, minced
- 2 bay leaves
- 1 teaspoon of thyme
- Salt and pepper to taste

Cooking Instructions:

1. In a large pot, combine chicken thighs, white rice, low-sodium chicken broth, sliced carrots, sliced celery, chopped onion, minced garlic, bay leaves, and thyme.
2. Bring to a boil, then reduce heat to simmer.
3. Cook for 30-35 minutes until chicken is cooked through and rice is tender.
4. Remove chicken thighs, shred them, and return to the pot.
5. Season with salt and pepper.

6. Serve hot.

Nutritional Information (per serving):

- Calories: 320
- Protein: 25g
- Carbohydrates: 35g
- Fiber: 2g
- Potassium: 320mg

TUNA SALAD

Benefit: High in protein, low in sodium and potassium.

- Prep Time: 15 minutes
- Servings: 2

Ingredients:

- 2 cans (5 ounces each) of low-sodium tuna, drained
- 1/2 cup of diced celery
- 1/4 cup of diced red onions
- 1/4 cup of low-fat mayonnaise
- 2 tablespoons of chopped fresh dill
- Juice of 1 lemon
- Salt and pepper to taste

Cooking Instructions:

1. In a bowl, combine drained tuna, diced celery, diced red onions, low-fat mayonnaise, chopped fresh dill, and lemon juice.
2. Season with salt and pepper.
3. Toss to combine.
4. Serve cold.

Nutritional Information (per serving):

- Calories: 220

- Protein: 25g
- Carbohydrates: 4g
- Fiber: 1g
- Potassium: 280mg

MINESTRONE SOUP

Benefit: High in fiber and flavor, low in sodium and potassium.

- Prep/Cook Time: 45 minutes
- Servings: 4

Ingredients:

- 1 cup of cooked small pasta (e.g., ditalini)
- 4 cups of low-sodium vegetable broth
- 1 can (15 ounces) of low-sodium kidney beans, drained and rinsed
- 1 cup of diced zucchini
- 1 cup of diced carrots
- 1 cup of diced celery
- 1 cup of diced tomatoes
- 1/2 cup of diced onions
- 2 cloves of garlic, minced
- 1 teaspoon of dried basil
- 1/2 teaspoon of dried oregano
- 1/4 cup of grated Parmesan cheese (low sodium)
- Salt and pepper to taste

Cooking Instructions:

1. In a large pot, combine low-sodium vegetable broth, drained kidney beans, diced zucchini, diced carrots, diced celery, diced tomatoes, diced onions, minced garlic, dried basil, and dried oregano.
2. Bring to a boil, then reduce heat to simmer.
3. Cook for 30-35 minutes until vegetables are tender.

4. Stir in cooked pasta.
5. Season with salt and pepper.
6. Serve hot, garnished with grated Parmesan cheese.

Nutritional Information (per serving):

- Calories: 320
- Protein: 13g
- Carbohydrates: 60g
- Fiber: 12g
- Potassium: 520mg

QUINOA AND BLACK BEAN SOUP

Benefit: High in protein and fiber, low in sodium and potassium.

- Prep/Cook Time: 40 minutes
- Servings: 4

Ingredients:

- 1 cup of cooked quinoa
- 4 cups of low-sodium vegetable broth
- 1 can (15 ounces) of low-sodium black beans, drained and rinsed
- 1 cup of diced tomatoes
- 1 cup of diced red onions
- 1 cup of diced bell peppers
- 2 cloves of garlic, minced
- 1 teaspoon of cumin
- 1/2 teaspoon of chili powder
- Juice of 1 lime
- 1/4 cup of chopped fresh cilantro
- Salt and pepper to taste

Cooking Instructions:

1. In a large pot, combine low-sodium vegetable broth, drained black beans, diced tomatoes, diced red onions, diced bell peppers, minced garlic, cumin, and chili powder.
2. Bring to a boil, then reduce heat to simmer.
3. Cook for 25-30 minutes.
4. Stir in cooked quinoa, lime juice, and chopped fresh cilantro.
5. Season with salt and pepper.
6. Serve hot.

Nutritional Information (per serving):

- Calories: 320
- Protein: 12g
- Carbohydrates: 55g
- Fiber: 13g
- Potassium: 540mg

SPINACH AND STRAWBERRY SALAD

Benefit: Low in sodium and potassium, a refreshing and nutrient-packed salad.

- Prep Time: 10 minutes
- Servings: 4

Ingredients:

- 6 cups of fresh baby spinach
- 2 cups of sliced strawberries
- 1/4 cup of chopped pecans
- 1/4 cup of crumbled feta cheese (low sodium)
- 2 tablespoons of balsamic vinaigrette dressing (low sodium)
- Salt and pepper to taste

Cooking Instructions:

1. In a large bowl, combine fresh baby spinach, sliced strawberries, chopped pecans, and crumbled feta cheese.
2. Drizzle with balsamic vinaigrette dressing.
3. Season with salt and pepper.
4. Toss to combine.
5. Serve cold.

Nutritional Information (per serving):

- Calories: 140
- Protein: 3g
- Carbohydrates: 15g
- Fiber: 4g
- Potassium: 330mg

BUTTERNUT SQUASH SOUP

Benefit: Low in sodium and potassium, a comforting and creamy soup.

- Prep/Cook Time: 1 hour
- Servings: 4

Ingredients:

- 1 butternut squash, peeled, seeded, and chopped
- 1 small onion, chopped
- 2 cloves of garlic, minced
- 4 cups of low-sodium vegetable broth
- 1/2 cup of low-fat sour cream
- 2 tablespoons of olive oil
- 1 teaspoon of dried sage
- Salt and pepper to taste

Cooking Instructions:

1. In a large pot, heat olive oil over medium heat.
2. Add chopped onion and minced garlic, sauté until softened.
3. Add chopped butternut squash and low-sodium vegetable broth.
4. Simmer for 30-35 minutes until squash is tender.
5. Use an immersion blender to blend until smooth.
6. Stir in low-fat sour cream and dried sage.
7. Season with salt and pepper. Serve hot.

Nutritional Information (per serving):

- Calories: 190
- Protein: 2g
- Carbohydrates: 25g
- Fiber: 5g
- Potassium: 560mg

CHICKPEA AND AVOCADO SALAD

Benefit: High in fiber and healthy fats, low in sodium and potassium.

- Prep Time: 10 minutes
- Servings: 4

Ingredients:

- 2 cans (15 ounces each) of low-sodium chickpeas, drained and rinsed
- 2 avocados, diced
- 1/2 cup of diced red onions
- 1/4 cup of chopped fresh cilantro
- Juice of 2 limes
- 2 tablespoons of extra-virgin olive oil
- Salt and pepper to taste

Cooking Instructions:

1. In a large bowl, combine drained chickpeas, diced avocados, diced red onions, and chopped fresh cilantro.
2. Drizzle with lime juice and extra-virgin olive oil.
3. Season with salt and pepper.
4. Toss to combine.
5. Serve cold.

Nutritional Information (per serving):

- Calories: 290
- Protein: 9g
- Carbohydrates: 27g
- Fiber: 11g
- Potassium: 570mg

TOMATO BASIL SOUP

Benefit: Low in sodium and potassium, a classic and flavorful soup.

- Prep/Cook Time: 30 minutes
- Servings: 4

Ingredients:

- 4 cups of low-sodium tomato juice
- 1 can (14 ounces) of diced tomatoes (no salt added)
- 1/2 cup of fresh basil leaves
- 2 cloves of garlic, minced
- 1/4 cup of low-fat milk
- 2 tablespoons of olive oil
- Salt and pepper to taste

Cooking Instructions:

1. In a blender, combine low-sodium tomato juice, diced tomatoes, fresh basil leaves, and minced garlic.
2. Blend until smooth.
3. Pour the mixture into a pot and heat over medium heat.
4. Stir in low-fat milk and olive oil.
5. Cook for 10-15 minutes until heated through.
6. Season with salt and pepper.
7. Serve hot.

Nutritional Information (per serving):

- Calories: 110
- Protein: 3g
- Carbohydrates: 15g
- Fiber: 3g
- Potassium: 450mg

CUCUMBER AND DILL SALAD

Benefit: Low in sodium and potassium, a refreshing and crunchy salad.

- Prep Time: 10 minutes
- Servings: 4

Ingredients:

- 2 cucumbers, sliced
- 1/4 cup of chopped fresh dill
- 1/4 cup of diced red onions
- 2 tablespoons of white vinegar
- 1 tablespoon of olive oil
- Salt and pepper to taste

Cooking Instructions:

1. In a large bowl, combine sliced cucumbers, chopped fresh dill, and diced red onions.
2. Drizzle with white vinegar and olive oil.
3. Season with salt and pepper.
4. Toss to combine.
5. Serve cold.

Nutritional Information (per serving):

- Calories: 40
- Protein: 1g
- Carbohydrates: 5g
- Fiber: 1g
- Potassium: 220mg

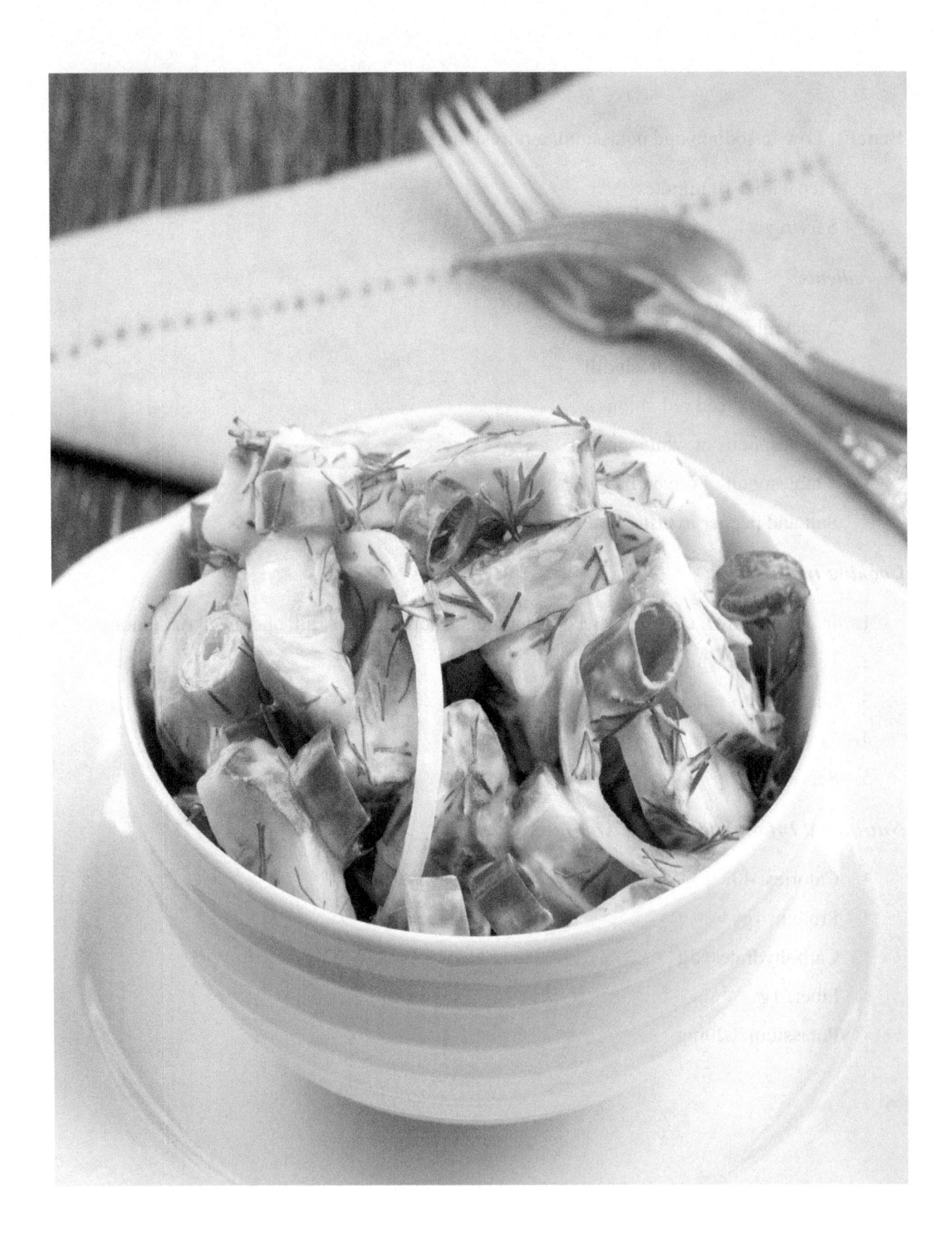

DESSERTS AND TREATS

BANANA ICE CREAM

Benefit: Low in sodium and potassium, a creamy and guilt-free dessert.

- Prep/Cook Time: 5 minutes
- Servings: 2

Ingredients:

- 2 ripe bananas, sliced and frozen
- 1/4 cup of unsweetened almond milk
- 1 teaspoon of vanilla extract
- Optional toppings: chopped nuts, dark chocolate chips (use sparingly)

Cooking Instructions:

1. Place frozen banana slices, almond milk, and vanilla extract in a blender or food processor.
2. Blend until smooth and creamy.
3. Serve immediately with your choice of optional toppings.

Nutritional Information (per serving):

- Calories: 90
- Protein: 1g
- Carbohydrates: 23g
- Fiber: 3g
- Potassium: 220mg

BAKED APPLES

Benefit: Low in sodium and potassium, a warm and comforting dessert.

- Prep/Cook Time: 45 minutes
- Servings: 4

Ingredients:

- 4 apples, cored and halved
- 1/4 cup of chopped walnuts
- 2 tablespoons of honey (use sparingly)
- 1 teaspoon of cinnamon
- 1/4 cup of water

Cooking Instructions:

1. Preheat the oven to 350°F (175°C).
2. In a small bowl, mix chopped walnuts, honey, and cinnamon.
3. Place apple halves in a baking dish and fill each with the walnut mixture.
4. Pour water into the baking dish.
5. Cover with foil and bake for 30-35 minutes, then uncover and bake for an additional 10 minutes until apples are tender.
6. Serve warm.

Nutritional Information (per serving):

- Calories: 150
- Protein: 2g
- Carbohydrates: 29g
- Fiber: 5g
- Potassium: 190mg

RICE PUDDING

Benefit: Creamy and low in sodium and potassium, a classic dessert.

- Prep/Cook Time: 1 hour
- Servings: 6

Ingredients:

- 1 cup of Arborio rice
- 4 cups of low-fat milk
- 1/4 cup of granulated sugar (use sparingly)

- 1 teaspoon of vanilla extract
- Ground cinnamon for garnish

Cooking Instructions:

1. In a large saucepan, combine Arborio rice, low-fat milk, and granulated sugar.
2. Bring to a boil, then reduce heat to low and simmer for 30-40 minutes, stirring frequently, until rice is tender and mixture thickens.
3. Stir in vanilla extract.
4. Remove from heat and let it cool.
5. Serve chilled, garnished with a sprinkle of ground cinnamon.

Nutritional Information (per serving):

- Calories: 250
- Protein: 7g
- Carbohydrates: 46g
- Fiber: 0g
- Potassium: 250mg

CHOCOLATE AVOCADO MOUSSE

Benefit: Low in sodium and potassium, a rich and indulgent dessert.

- Prep/Cook Time: 15 minutes
- Servings: 4

Ingredients:

- 2 ripe avocados
- 1/4 cup of unsweetened cocoa powder
- 1/4 cup of honey (use sparingly)
- 1 teaspoon of vanilla extract

Cooking Instructions:

1. Scoop the flesh of the avocados into a blender or food processor.
2. Add cocoa powder, honey, and vanilla extract.

3. Blend until smooth and creamy.
4. Chill in the refrigerator for at least 30 minutes before serving.

Nutritional Information (per serving):

- Calories: 220
- Protein: 3g
- Carbohydrates: 29g
- Fiber: 7g
- Potassium: 510mg

OATMEAL RAISIN COOKIES

Benefit: Low in sodium and potassium, a wholesome cookie option.

- Prep/Cook Time: 25 minutes
- Servings: 12

Ingredients:

- 1 cup of old-fashioned oats
- 1/2 cup of whole wheat flour
- 1/2 cup of raisins
- 1/4 cup of unsalted butter, softened
- 1/4 cup of honey (use sparingly)
- 1 egg
- 1/2 teaspoon of cinnamon
- 1/2 teaspoon of vanilla extract
- 1/4 teaspoon of baking soda

Cooking Instructions:

1. Preheat the oven to 350°F (175°C) and line a baking sheet with parchment paper.
2. In a mixing bowl, combine softened butter, honey, egg, and vanilla extract.
3. In a separate bowl, mix oats, whole wheat flour, raisins, cinnamon, and baking soda.
4. Combine the wet and dry ingredients and mix until well incorporated.

5. Drop spoonfuls of cookie dough onto the prepared baking sheet.
6. Bake for 12-15 minutes until the edges are golden.
7. Let the cookies cool on a wire rack before serving.

Nutritional Information (per serving - 1 cookie):

- Calories: 120
- Protein: 2g
- Carbohydrates: 18g
- Fiber: 2g
- Potassium: 45mg

BERRY PARFAIT

Benefit: Low in sodium and potassium, a refreshing and colorful dessert.

- Prep Time: 10 minutes
- Servings: 2

Ingredients:

- 1 cup of low-fat Greek yogurt
- 1/2 cup of mixed berries (e.g., strawberries, blueberries, raspberries)
- 2 tablespoons of honey (use sparingly)
- 2 tablespoons of granola (low sodium)

Cooking Instructions:

1. In two serving glasses, layer low-fat Greek yogurt, mixed berries, and honey.
2. Repeat the layers until the glasses are filled.
3. Top with granola for added crunch.
4. Serve chilled.

Nutritional Information (per serving):

- Calories: 180
- Protein: 12g
- Carbohydrates: 32g

- Fiber: 3g
- Potassium: 230mg

PINEAPPLE SORBET

Benefit: Low in sodium and potassium, a tropical and refreshing dessert.

- Prep/Cook Time: 10 minutes
- Servings: 4

Ingredients:

- 4 cups of frozen pineapple chunks
- 1/4 cup of unsweetened coconut milk
- 2 tablespoons of honey (use sparingly)
- Juice of 1 lime

Cooking Instructions:

1. Place frozen pineapple chunks, coconut milk, honey, and lime juice in a blender or food processor.
2. Blend until smooth and creamy.
3. Serve immediately or freeze for a firmer texture.

Nutritional Information (per serving):

- Calories: 110
- Protein: 1g
- Carbohydrates: 29g
- Fiber: 3g
- Potassium: 160mg

LEMON BARS

Benefit: Low in sodium and potassium, a zesty and sweet dessert.

- Prep/Cook Time: 40 minutes
- Servings: 12

Ingredients:

For the crust:

- 1 cup of almond flour
- 2 tablespoons of coconut oil, melted
- 2 tablespoons of honey (use sparingly)

For the lemon filling:

- 3 large eggs
- 1/2 cup of fresh lemon juice
- Zest of 1 lemon
- 1/4 cup of honey (use sparingly)
- 1/4 cup of almond flour
- 1/2 teaspoon of baking powder
- Powdered sugar for dusting (optional)

Cooking Instructions:

1. Preheat the oven to 350°F (175°C) and line an 8x8-inch baking dish with parchment paper.
2. In a bowl, mix almond flour, melted coconut oil, and honey to make the crust.
3. Press the crust mixture into the bottom of the prepared baking dish.
4. Bake for 10-12 minutes until lightly golden.
5. In another bowl, whisk together eggs, fresh lemon juice, lemon zest, honey, almond flour, and baking powder to make the lemon filling.
6. Pour the lemon filling over the baked crust.
7. Bake for an additional 20-25 minutes until the filling is set.
8. Let it cool, then refrigerate until firm.
9. Dust with powdered sugar if desired before serving.

Nutritional Information (per serving):

- Calories: 150
- Protein: 3g
- Carbohydrates: 15g
- Fiber: 1g
- Potassium: 65mg

FROZEN YOGURT BITES

Benefit: Low in sodium and potassium, a simple and satisfying treat.

- Prep/Cook Time: 2 hours (includes freezing time)
- Servings: 4

Ingredients:

- 1 cup of low-fat vanilla yogurt
- 1/2 cup of fresh strawberries, diced
- 1/2 cup of fresh blueberries
- 2 tablespoons of honey (use sparingly)

Cooking Instructions:

1. In a bowl, mix low-fat vanilla yogurt and honey until well combined.
2. Line a mini muffin tin with silicone molds or paper liners.
3. Spoon a small amount of the yogurt mixture into each mold, filling them about halfway.
4. Add diced strawberries and blueberries on top of the yogurt.
5. Top with more yogurt to cover the berries.
6. Freeze for at least 2 hours until the bites are firm.
7. Pop the bites out of the molds and serve frozen.

Nutritional Information (per serving):

- Calories: 70
- Protein: 3g
- Carbohydrates: 15g
- Fiber: 1g
- Potassium: 100mg

CHOCOLATE-COVERED STRAWBERRIES

Benefit: Low in sodium and potassium, a decadent and romantic dessert.

- Prep/Cook Time: 20 minutes
- Servings: 4

Ingredients:

- 12 fresh strawberries, washed and dried
- 3 ounces of dark chocolate (70% cocoa or higher), chopped
- 1 teaspoon of coconut oil
- Chopped nuts (optional topping)

Cooking Instructions:

1. In a microwave-safe bowl, combine chopped dark chocolate and coconut oil.
2. Microwave in 20-second intervals, stirring between each interval, until the chocolate is melted and smooth.
3. Dip each strawberry into the melted chocolate, allowing any excess to drip off.
4. Place the chocolate-covered strawberries on a parchment paper-lined tray.
5. If desired, sprinkle with chopped nuts while the chocolate is still soft.
6. Let them cool and harden in the refrigerator for about 30 minutes.
7. Serve chilled.

Nutritional Information (per serving - 3 strawberries):

- Calories: 160
- Protein: 2g
- Carbohydrates: 20g
- Fiber: 3g
- Potassium: 130mg

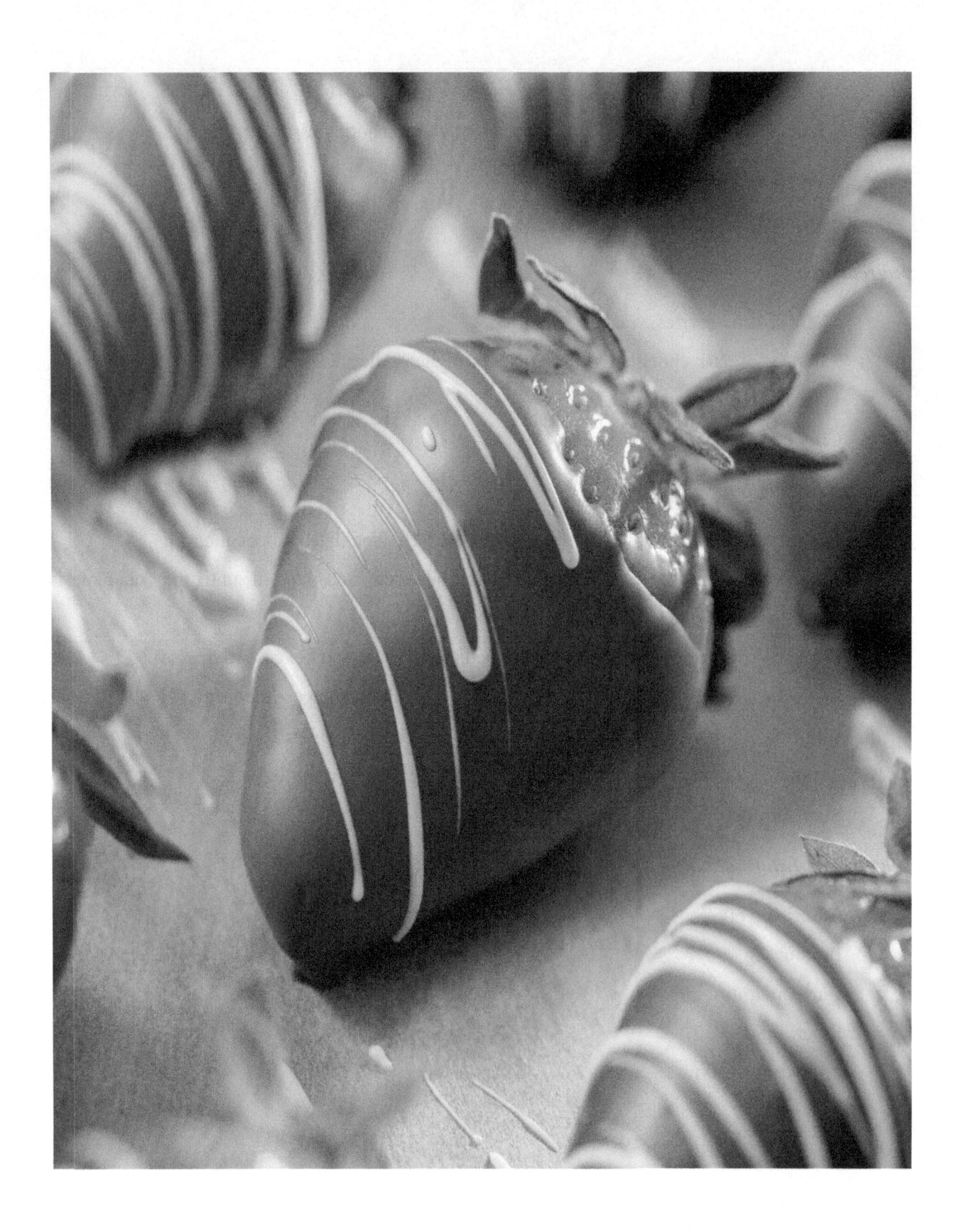

BEVERAGES

HERBAL TEAS FOR KIDNEY SUPPORT

DANDELION ROOT TEA

Benefit: Supports kidney function and detoxification.

- Prep Time: 5 minutes
- Servings: 2

Ingredients:

- 2 teaspoons of dried dandelion root
- 2 cups of boiling water

Instructions:

1. Place dried dandelion root in a teapot or heatproof container.
2. Pour boiling water over the dandelion root.
3. Cover and steep for 10-15 minutes.
4. Strain and serve. You can sweeten it with honey if desired.

Nutritional Information (per serving):

- Calories: 0
- Protein: 0g
- Carbohydrates: 0g
- Fiber: 0g
- Potassium: 0mg

NETTLE LEAF TEA

Benefit: Supports kidney health and may help reduce fluid retention.

- Prep Time: 5 minutes
- Servings: 2

Ingredients:

- 2 teaspoons of dried nettle leaves
- 2 cups of boiling water

Instructions:

1. Place dried nettle leaves in a teapot or heatproof container.
2. Pour boiling water over the nettle leaves.
3. Cover and steep for 5-10 minutes.
4. Strain and serve.

Nutritional Information (per serving):

- Calories: 0
- Protein: 0g
- Carbohydrates: 0g
- Fiber: 0g
- Potassium: 0mg

HIBISCUS TEA

Benefit: May help lower blood pressure and provide antioxidants.

- Prep Time: 5 minutes
- Servings: 2

Ingredients:

- 2 teaspoons of dried hibiscus flowers
- 2 cups of boiling water
- Honey or stevia (use sparingly) for sweetness (optional)

Instructions:

1. Place dried hibiscus flowers in a teapot or heatproof container.
2. Pour boiling water over the hibiscus flowers.
3. Cover and steep for 5-10 minutes.
4. Strain and sweeten with honey or stevia if desired.

Nutritional Information (per serving):

- Calories: 0
- Protein: 0g
- Carbohydrates: 0g
- Fiber: 0g
- Potassium: 0mg

GINGER TEA

Benefit: May help reduce inflammation and support digestion.

- Prep Time: 10 minutes
- Servings: 2

Ingredients:

- 1-inch piece of fresh ginger, sliced
- 2 cups of water
- Honey or lemon (use sparingly) for flavor (optional)

Instructions:

1. In a saucepan, bring water to a boil.
2. Add sliced ginger and simmer for 5-10 minutes.
3. Remove from heat, strain, and add honey or lemon for flavor if desired.
4. Serve hot.

Nutritional Information (per serving):

- Calories: 0
- Protein: 0g
- Carbohydrates: 0g
- Fiber: 0g
- Potassium: 0mg

PARSLEY TEA

Benefit: May support kidney health and act as a diuretic.

- Prep Time: 10 minutes
- Servings: 2

Ingredients:

- 2 teaspoons of dried parsley leaves
- 2 cups of boiling water

Instructions:

1. Place dried parsley leaves in a teapot or heatproof container.
2. Pour boiling water over the parsley leaves.
3. Cover and steep for 10 minutes.
4. Strain and serve.

Nutritional Information (per serving):

- Calories: 0
- Protein: 0g
- Carbohydrates: 0g
- Fiber: 0g
- Potassium: 0mg

LOW POTASSIUM-INFUSED WATER

CUCUMBER AND MINT INFUSED WATER

Benefit: Refreshing and low in potassium.

- Prep Time: 5 minutes
- Servings: 4

Ingredients:

- 1 cucumber, sliced
- 8-10 fresh mint leaves
- 4 cups of water

Instructions:

1. Place cucumber slices and mint leaves in a pitcher.
2. Add water and stir.
3. Refrigerate for at least an hour to infuse the flavors.
4. Serve over ice.

Nutritional Information (per serving):

- Calories: 0
- Protein: 0g
- Carbohydrates: 0g
- Fiber: 0g
- Potassium: 40mg

LEMON AND LIME INFUSED WATER

Benefit: Hydrating and low in potassium.

- Prep Time: 5 minutes
- Servings: 4

Ingredients:

- 1 lemon, sliced
- 1 lime, sliced
- 4 cups of water

Instructions:

1. Place lemon and lime slices in a pitcher.
2. Add water and stir.
3. Refrigerate for at least an hour to infuse the citrus flavors.
4. Serve over ice.

Nutritional Information (per serving):

- Calories: 0
- Protein: 0g
- Carbohydrates: 0g
- Fiber: 0g
- Potassium: 60mg

BERRY BLAST INFUSED WATER

Benefit: Delicious and low in potassium.

- Prep Time: 5 minutes
- Servings: 4

Ingredients:

- 1 cup of mixed berries (e.g., strawberries, blueberries, raspberries)
- 4 cups of water

Instructions:

1. Mash the mixed berries slightly to release their flavor.
2. Place mashed berries in a pitcher.
3. Add water and stir.
4. Refrigerate for at least an hour to infuse the berry flavors.
5. Serve over ice.

Nutritional Information (per serving):

- Calories: 15
- Protein: 0g
- Carbohydrates: 4g
- Fiber: 2g
- Potassium: 70mg

PEACH AND BASIL INFUSED WATER

Benefit: Refreshing and low in potassium.

- Prep Time: 5 minutes
- Servings: 4

Ingredients:

2 peaches, sliced

8-10 fresh basil leaves

4 cups of water

Instructions:

1. Place peach slices and basil leaves in a pitcher.
2. Add water and stir.
3. Refrigerate for at least an hour to infuse the flavors.
4. Serve over ice.

Nutritional Information (per serving):

- Calories: 20
- Protein: 0g
- Carbohydrates: 5g
- Fiber: 1g
- Potassium: 140mg

HOMEMADE ELECTROLYTE DRINKS

DIY ELECTROLYTE SOLUTION

Benefit: Replenishes electrolytes lost during kidney issues or dialysis.

- Prep Time: 5 minutes
- Servings: 2

Ingredients:

- 2 cups of water
- 1/2 teaspoon of salt (use sparingly)
- 1 tablespoon of honey (use sparingly)
- 1/4 cup of orange juice (optional)

Instructions:

1. Mix water, salt, honey, and orange juice (if using) in a pitcher.
2. Stir until salt and honey are dissolved.
3. Serve chilled.

Nutritional Information (per serving):

- Calories: 40 (without orange juice)
- Protein: 0g
- Carbohydrates: 11g (without orange juice)
- Fiber: 0g
- Potassium: 200mg (without orange juice)

GREEN TEA ELECTROLYTE COOLER

Benefit: Provides electrolytes and antioxidants.

- Prep Time: 10 minutes
- Servings: 2

Ingredients:

- 2 green tea bags
- 2 cups of water
- 1/4 teaspoon of salt (use sparingly)
- 2 tablespoons of honey (use sparingly)
- Juice of 1/2 lemon

Instructions:

- Steep green tea bags in boiling water for 3-5 minutes.
- Remove tea bags and let it cool to room temperature.
- Mix in salt, honey, and lemon juice.
- Refrigerate until chilled.
- Serve over ice.

Nutritional Information (per serving):

- Calories: 60
- Protein: 0g
- Carbohydrates: 16g
- Fiber: 0g
- Potassium: 70mg

PINEAPPLE COCONUT ELECTROLYTE SMOOTHIE

Benefit: Hydrating and provides electrolytes.

- Prep Time: 10 minutes
- Servings: 2

Ingredients:

- 1 cup of fresh pineapple chunks
- 1/2 cup of coconut water
- 1/4 teaspoon of salt (use sparingly)
- 2 tablespoons of honey (use sparingly)
- 1/2 cup of ice cubes

Instructions:

1. Blend fresh pineapple chunks and coconut water until smooth.
2. Add salt, honey, and ice cubes.
3. Blend again until well mixed and frothy.
4. Serve immediately.

Nutritional Information (per serving):

- Calories: 120
- Protein: 1g
- Carbohydrates: 31g
- Fiber: 2g
- Potassium: 240mg

WATERMELON AND MINT ELECTROLYTE REFRESHER

Benefit: Hydrating and replenishes electrolytes.

- Prep Time: 10 minutes
- Servings: 2

Ingredients:

- 2 cups of watermelon, cubed and seeded
- 1/2 cup of coconut water
- 1/4 teaspoon of salt (use sparingly)
- 1 tablespoon of honey (use sparingly)
- Fresh mint leaves for garnish

Instructions:

1. Place watermelon cubes and coconut water in a blender.
2. Blend until smooth.
3. Add salt and honey, then blend again until well mixed.
4. Serve chilled, garnished with fresh mint leaves.

Nutritional Information (per serving):

- Calories: 90
- Protein: 1g
- Carbohydrates: 23g
- Fiber: 1g
- Potassium: 360mg

COCONUT WATER ELECTROLYTE DRINK

Benefit: Provides natural electrolytes and hydration.

- Prep Time: 5 minutes
- Servings: 2

Ingredients:

- 2 cups of coconut water
- 1/4 teaspoon of salt (use sparingly)
- 2 tablespoons of honey (use sparingly)
- Juice of 1/2 lime

Instructions:

1. Mix coconut water, salt, honey, and lime juice in a pitcher.
2. Stir until salt and honey are dissolved.
3. Serve chilled.

Nutritional Information (per serving):

- Calories: 80
- Protein: 1g
- Carbohydrates: 20g
- Fiber: 0g
- Potassium: 600mg

WATERMELON ELECTROLYTE COOLER

Benefit: Refreshing and replenishes electrolytes.

- Prep Time: 10 minutes
- Servings: 4

Ingredients:

- 4 cups of watermelon, cubed and seeded
- 1/4 teaspoon of salt (use sparingly)
- 1 tablespoon of honey (use sparingly)
- Juice of 1/2 lemon

Instructions:

1. Place watermelon cubes in a blender and blend until smooth.
2. Strain the watermelon puree to remove seeds and pulp.
3. Mix watermelon juice, salt, honey, and lemon juice in a pitcher.
4. Stir until salt and honey are dissolved.
5. Serve chilled.

Nutritional Information (per serving):

- Calories: 50
- Protein: 1g
- Carbohydrates: 13g
- Fiber: 1g
- Potassium: 170mg

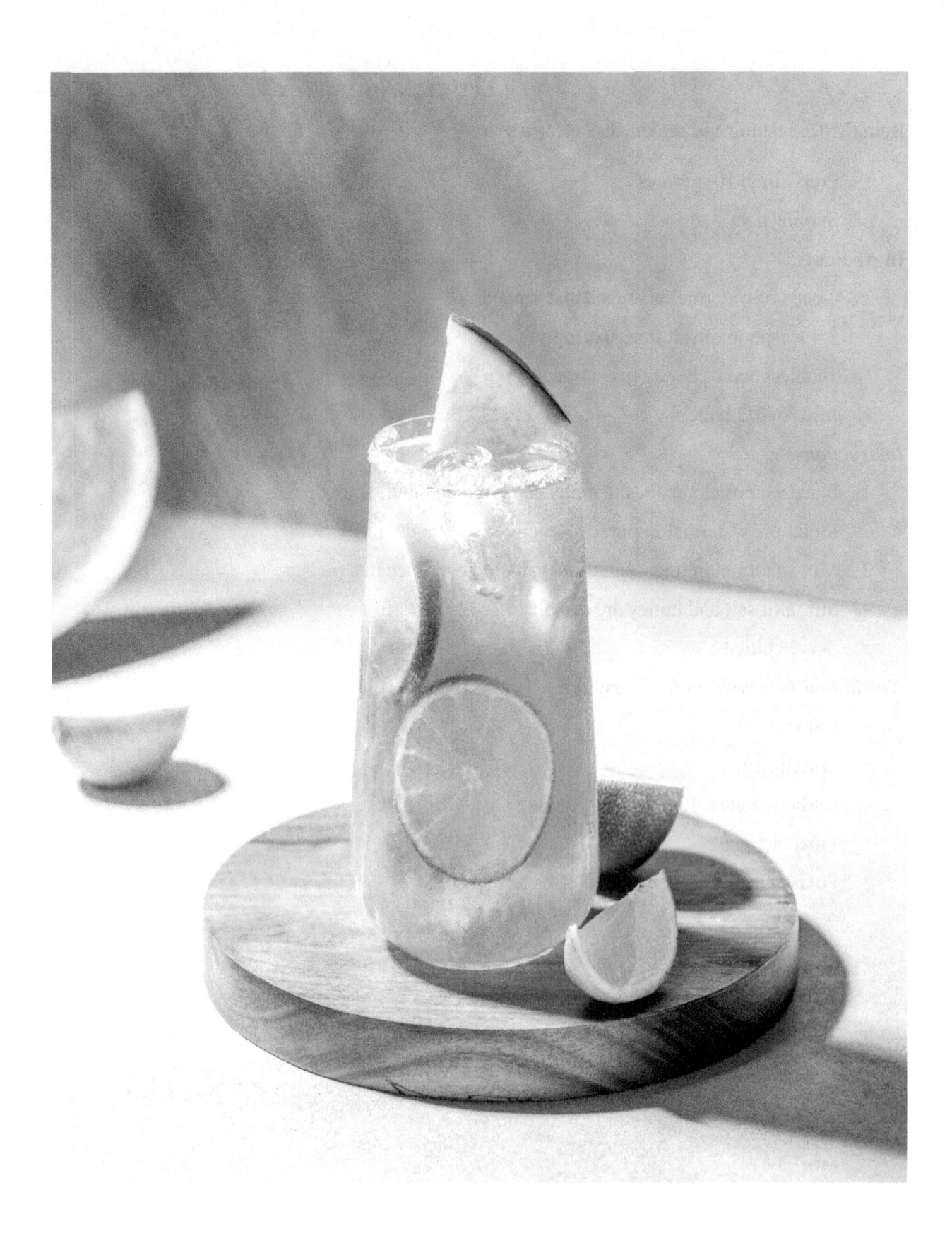

CHAPTER TWO: 30-DAY MEAL PLAN AND GROCERY SHOPPING GUIDE

Day	Breakfast	Lunch	Dinner	Snack	Dessert	Beverage
1	Creamy Oatmeal with Blueberries	Mediterranean Quinoa Salad	Lemon Herb Baked Chicken with Roasted Vegetables	Cucumber and Hummus	Baked Apples with Cinnamon	Herbal Tea
2	Scrambled Eggs with Spinach and Tomatoes	Chickpea and Vegetable Stir-Fry	Baked Salmon with Dill and Asparagus	Greek Yogurt with Berries	Frozen Banana Bites	Low Potassium-Infused Water
3	Banana and Almond Smoothie	Lentil and Vegetable Soup	Turkey and Vegetable Kebabs	Rice Cakes with Nut Butter	Chia Seed Pudding	Homemade Electrolyte Drink
4	Quinoa Breakfast Bowl with Sliced Peaches	Spinach and Strawberry Salad with Vinaigrette	Grilled Whitefish with Lemon Butter Sauce and Steamed Broccoli	Sliced Cucumber with Tzatziki	Berry Sorbet	Herbal Tea
5	Greek Yogurt Parfait with Granola and Berries	Caprese Salad with Low-Sodium Mozzarella	Baked Chicken Breast with Garlic Mashed Cauliflower	Carrot Sticks with Hummus	Baked Pears with Honey and Cinnamon	Low Potassium-Infused Water
6	Spinach and Feta Omelette	Quinoa and Black Bean Salad	Lemon Garlic Shrimp with Asparagus and Quinoa	Sliced Apples with Almond Butter	Mango Sorbet	Homemade Electrolyte Drink
7	Creamy Banana and Peanut Butter Smoothie	Roasted Vegetable Wrap with Hummus	Beef Stir-Fry with Bok Choy and Brown Rice	Cottage Cheese with Pineapple	Baked Peaches with a Drizzle of Honey	Herbal Tea
8	Whole Grain Pancakes with Fresh Berries	Tuna Salad Lettuce Wraps	Baked Salmon with Dill Sauce	Sliced Apple with Almond Butter	Apple and Cinnamon Rice Pudding	Low Potassium-Infused Water

9	Veggie and Cheese Breakfast Burrito	Greek Salad with Grilled Chicken	Mediterranean Quinoa Salad	Cottage Cheese with Sliced Strawberries	Baked Bananas with Walnuts and Honey	Herbal Tea
10	Creamy Coconut Chia Pudding	Lemon Garlic Shrimp and Asparagus	Stir-Fried Tofu with Broccoli and Brown Rice	Sliced Peppers and Cherry Tomatoes with Hummus	Blueberry and Almond Bites	Homemade Electrolyte Drink
11	Quinoa Breakfast Bowl with Sliced Peaches	Tomato Basil Soup	Spinach and Strawberry Salad	Sliced Cucumber with Tzatziki	Baked Pears with Honey and Cinnamon	Low Potassium-Infused Water
12	Rice Cake with Peanut Butter and Banana	Lemon Herb Baked Salmon	Chickpea and Vegetable Curry with Brown Rice	Sliced Apples with Almond Butter	Mixed Berry Sorbet	Herbal Tea
13	Scrambled Eggs with Sautéed Spinach and Tomatoes	Lentil and Vegetable Soup	Grilled with Lemon Herb Chicken	Rice Cakes with Nut Butter	Chia Seed Pudding	Homemade Electrolyte Drink
14	Banana and Almond Smoothie	Mediterranean Quinoa Salad	Turkey and Vegetable Stir-Fry with Brown Rice	Greek Yogurt with Berries	Frozen Banana Bites	Low Potassium-Infused Water
15	Creamy Oatmeal with Blueberries	Spinach and Strawberry Salad	Lemon Garlic Shrimp with Asparagus and Quinoa	Sliced Bell Peppers with Guacamole	Baked Apples with Cinnamon	Herbal Tea
16	Greek Yogurt Parfait with Granola and Berries	Tuna Salad Lettuce Wraps	Baked Salmon with Dill Sauce	Cucumber and Hummus	Baked Peaches with a Drizzle of Honey	Low Potassium-Infused Water

17	Whole Grain Pancakes with Fresh Berries	Caprese Salad with Low-Sodium Mozzarella	Pork Tenderloin with Herb Roasted Potatoes and Grilled Asparagus	Sliced Strawberries with Cottage Cheese	Blueberry and Almond Bites	Homemade Electrolyte Drink
18	Veggie and Cheese Breakfast Burrito (Use low-sodium cheese)	Quinoa and Black Bean Salad	Beef Stir-Fry with Bok Choy and Brown Rice	Sliced Carrots with Hummus	Mango Sorbet	Herbal Tea
19	Creamy Coconut Chia Pudding	Chickpea and Vegetable Stir-Fry with Brown Rice	Grilled Whitefish with Lemon Butter Sauce and Roasted Brussels Sprouts	Sliced Apples with Almond Butter	Chia Seed Pudding	Low Potassium-Infused Water
20	Fruit and Nut Breakfast Quinoa	Mediterranean Quinoa Salad	Lemon Herb Baked Salmon with Steamed Broccoli	Rice Cakes with Nut Butter	Mixed Berry Sorbet	Herbal Tea
21	Quinoa Breakfast Bowl with Sliced Peaches	Lentil and Vegetable Soup	Turkey and Vegetable Kebabs with Garlic Mashed Cauliflower	Greek Yogurt with Berries	Frozen Banana Bites	Homemade Electrolyte Drink
22	Creamy Oatmeal with Blueberries	Spinach and Strawberry Salad with Balsamic Vinaigrette	Lemon Garlic Shrimp with Asparagus and Quinoa	Sliced Bell Peppers with Guacamole	Baked Apples with Cinnamon	Herbal Tea
23	Greek Yogurt Parfait with Granola and Berries	Tuna Salad Lettuce Wraps	Baked Chicken Breast with Garlic	Cucumber and Hummus	Baked Peaches with a Drizzle of Honey	Low Potassium-Infused Water
24	Whole Grain Pancakes	Caprese Salad with Low-	Beef Stir-Fry with Bok	Sliced Strawberries with	Blueberry and	Homemade Electrolyte Drink

	with Fresh Berries	Sodium Mozzarella	Choy and Brown Rice	Cottage Cheese	Almond Bites	
25	Veggie and Cheese Breakfast Burrito (Use low-sodium cheese)	Quinoa and Black Bean Salad	Lemon Garlic Shrimp with Asparagus and Quinoa	Sliced Carrots with Hummus	Mango Sorbet	Herbal Tea
26	Creamy Coconut Chia Pudding	Chickpea and Vegetable Stir-Fry with Brown Rice	Grilled Whitefish with Lemon Butter Sauce and Roasted Brussels Sprouts	Sliced Apples with Almond Butter	Chia Seed Pudding	Low Potassium-Infused Water
27	Fruit and Nut Breakfast Quinoa	Mediterranean Quinoa Salad	Lemon Herb Baked Salmon with Steamed Broccoli	Rice Cakes with Nut Butter	Mixed Berry Sorbet	Herbal Tea
28	Green Smoothie with Kale, Banana, and Almond Milk	Lentil and Vegetable Soup	Turkey and Vegetable Kebabs with Garlic Mashed Cauliflower	Greek Yogurt with Berries	Frozen Banana Bites	Homemade Electrolyte Drink
29	Creamy Oatmeal with Blueberries	Spinach and Strawberry Salad with Balsamic Vinaigrette	Lemon Garlic Shrimp with Asparagus and Quinoa	Sliced Bell Peppers with Guacamole	Baked Apples with Cinnamon	Herbal Tea
30	Greek Yogurt Parfait with Granola and Berries	Tuna Salad Lettuce Wraps	Baked Chicken Breast with Garlic Mashed Cauliflower and Steamed Green Beans	Cucumber and Hummus	Baked Peaches with a Drizzle of Honey	Low Potassium-Infused Water

Feel free to repeat these meal combinations in any order you prefer to complete your 30-day meal plan. Adapt portion sizes and dietary restrictions as necessary based on individual needs and guidance from a healthcare provider or registered dietitian. This comprehensive plan offers a diverse range of kidney-friendly recipes to support your journey in managing Stage 3 Kidney Disease effectively while enjoying delicious, nutritious meals.

GROCERY SHOPPING GUIDE

Managing your diet is crucial when you have Stage 3 Kidney Disease, also known as Chronic Kidney Disease (CKD). A kidney-friendly diet can help slow the progression of the disease and reduce complications. Here's a grocery shopping guide to help you make healthier choices while adhering to your dietary restrictions:

1. Lean Proteins

- Skinless poultry (chicken or turkey)
- Lean cuts of beef or pork
- Fish (salmon, trout, tuna, or whitefish)
- Eggs

2. Low-Potassium Fruits

- Apples
- Berries (strawberries, blueberries, raspberries)
- Pineapple
- Cranberries
- Red grapes

3. Low-Potassium Vegetables

- Cabbage
- Cauliflower
- Bell peppers (red, green, or yellow)
- Onions
- Green beans

4. Low-Potassium Starches

- White rice
- White bread
- Pasta

- Cornflakes or rice cereal
- Flour tortillas

5. Dairy and Dairy Alternatives

- Low-fat or fat-free milk
- Low-fat yogurt
- Low-fat cheese (in moderation)
- Dairy-free milk alternatives (almond, rice, or oat milk)

6. Snacks and Condiments

- Unsalted popcorn
- Rice cakes
- Low-sodium crackers
- Mustard or vinegar-based salad dressings
- Unsalted nut butter (in moderation)

7. Beverages

- Water
- Herbal teas (e.g., chamomile, ginger, hibiscus)
- Low-potassium fruit juices (apple or cranberry)
- Homemade electrolyte drinks (as mentioned in previous recipes)

8. Canned or Frozen Foods (choose low-sodium options)

- Canned fruits (in juice, not syrup)
- Canned vegetables (rinsed to reduce sodium)
- Frozen vegetables (without added sauces)
- Frozen berries (for smoothies)

9. Cooking Ingredients

- Olive oil
- Herbs and spices (to flavor food without salt)

- Low-sodium broths or stocks
- Cornstarch (for thickening sauces)
- Low-sodium soy sauce (use sparingly)

10. Limit or Avoid

- High-potassium fruits and vegetables (bananas, oranges, potatoes, spinach)
- Processed and salty foods (chips, canned soups, fast food)
- High-sodium condiments (soy sauce, ketchup, barbecue sauce)
- Full-fat dairy products
- Nuts and seeds (in moderation)

11. Meal Planning

- Plan your meals to ensure a balanced diet.
- Control portion sizes to manage potassium and phosphorus intake.
- Monitor your fluid intake to prevent dehydration.

12. Consult a Dietitian

- Consider working with a registered dietitian specializing in kidney disease to create a personalized meal plan.
- They can help you navigate dietary restrictions and make the best food choices for your specific needs.

13. Read Labels

- Pay attention to nutrition labels to check for sodium, potassium, and phosphorus content.

14. Stay Hydrated

- Drink water in moderation, following your healthcare provider's recommendations.

Monitor Your Lab Results

Regularly check your kidney function and nutrient levels through blood tests. Adjust your diet as needed based on your results.

Remember that dietary recommendations can vary from person to person, so it's essential to consult with your healthcare provider or a registered dietitian who can provide tailored advice and guidance based on your individual health and stage of kidney disease. This grocery shopping guide is a general overview to help you get started on a kidney-friendly diet for Stage 3 Kidney Disease.

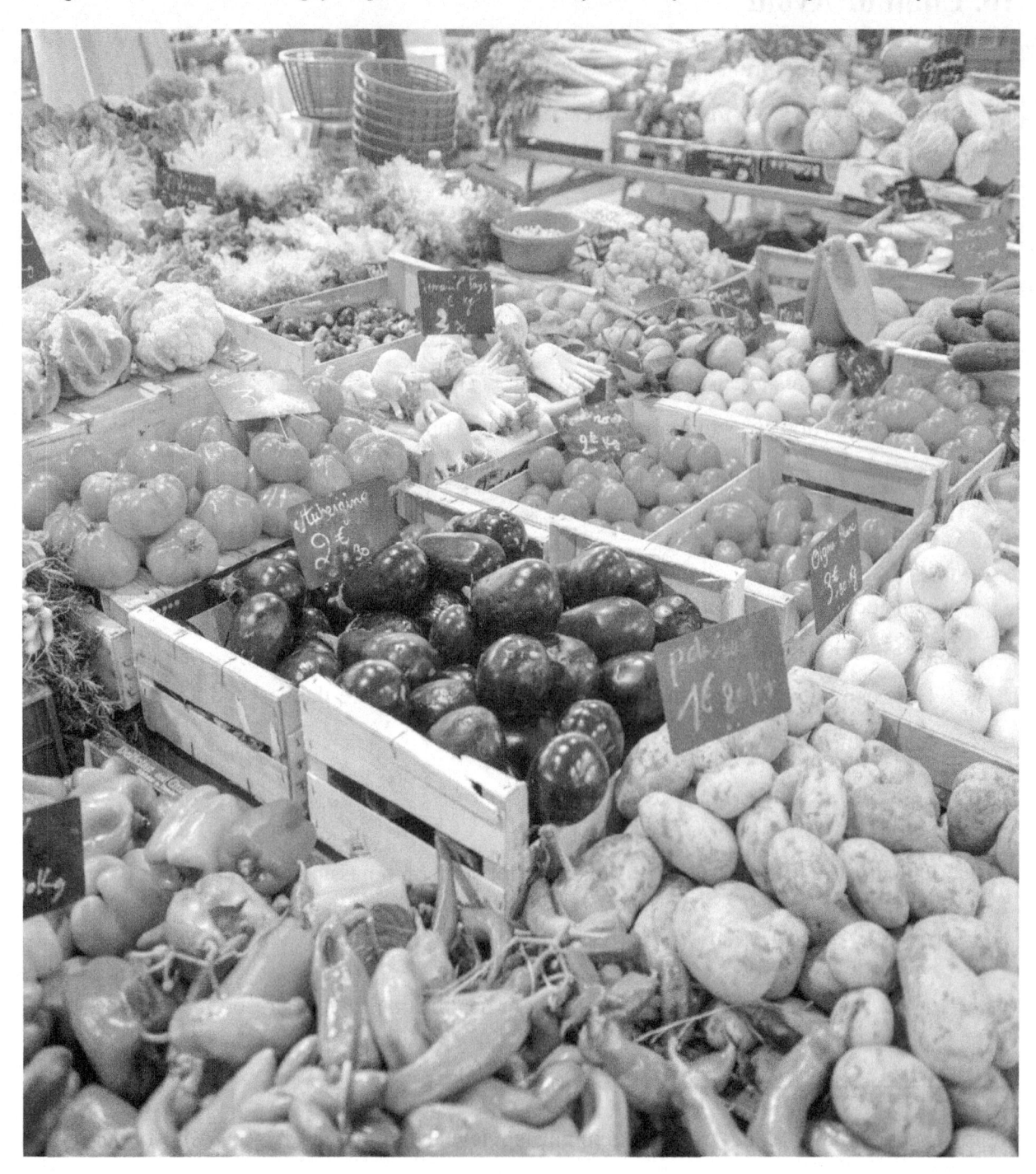

CONCLUSION

As we near the end of our journey through the Kidney Disease Diet Cookbook for Stage 3, it's important to consider the wonderful impact that diet can have on our health, especially when dealing with the problems of Chronic Kidney Disease (CKD). This cookbook was created with the concept that controlling Stage 3 Kidney Disease is about embracing a lifestyle that nourishes your kidneys and fosters your whole well-being.

Throughout this cookbook, we have looked at the causes, symptoms, and risk factors associated with kidney disease. Knowledge is power, understanding your situation is the first step toward regaining control of your health. With this knowledge, you can collaborate with your healthcare team to make informed decisions that benefit your kidney health.

We have looked at how nutrition can help you manage Stage 3 Kidney Disease. Your everyday food choices can slow the progression of CKD, alleviate symptoms, and improve your overall quality of life. By following the kidney-friendly recipes and meal plans provided, you're not just eating; you're actively managing your condition.

One of the most notable aspects of this cookbook is the sheer variety and flavor it offers. Kidney-friendly eating does not have to be bland. These recipes, which range from hearty breakfasts to filling main courses and scrumptious desserts, are intended to excite your taste buds while keeping to the dietary requirements for CKD.

We understand that each person's journey with kidney disease is unique. Your dietary requirements may differ from those of others due to conditions such as diabetes, hypertension, or personal preferences. As a result, we recommend consulting with a trained dietitian or healthcare provider to personalize your nutrition plan to your unique needs.

This cookbook invites you to embrace a holistic approach to wellness in addition to eating. Staying hydrated, stress management and physical activity are all essential components of your kidney health journey. We've included recipes for refreshing beverages, grocery shopping guidance, and tips for reading food labels, all with the objective of supporting your wellness goals.

Remember that you are not alone on this journey. Seek the help of family and friends, and consider joining kidney disease support groups or online communities where you can share your experiences and learn from others who are going through similar things.

Finally, the Kidney Disease Diet Cookbook for Stage 3 is more than simply a cookbook; it's a step-by-step guide to living a kidney-friendly lifestyle. You are taking big strides toward improving your well-being and thriving despite the obstacles of CKD by making conscientious eating choices, controlling your health, and nurturing your kidneys. Your journey exemplifies resilience, and we are here to help you every step of the way. May this cookbook be a helpful guide on your journey to greater kidney health and a brighter future.

MEAL PLANNING JOURNAL

KIDNEY DIET
Meal Planner

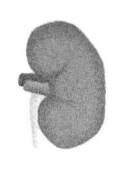

	BREAKFAST	LUNCH	DINNER
MON			
TUE			
WED			
THU			
FRI			
SAT			
SUN			

Your strength shines brightest in the face of adversity.
Keep shining; you are a beacon of hope

Date:

Shopping List

Note:

KIDNEY DIET
Meal Planner

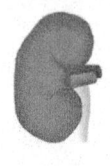

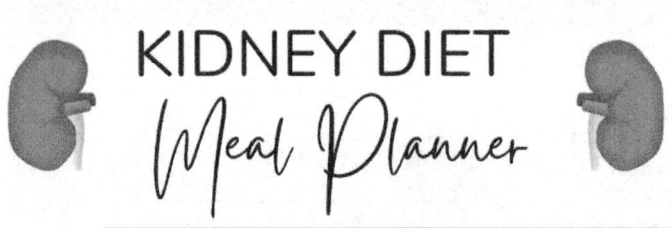

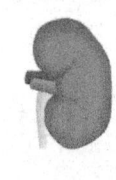

	BREAKFAST	LUNCH	DINNER
MON			
TUE			
WED			
THU			
FRI			
SAT			
SUN			

Your health is a reflection of the choices you make every day. Choose wisely, and you'll create a brighter future.

Date: ....

Shopping List

Note:

KIDNEY DIET
Meal Planner

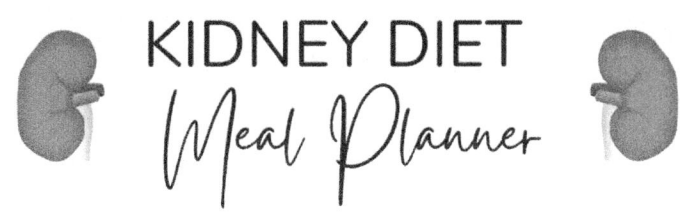

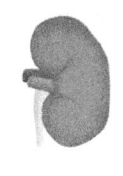

	BREAKFAST	LUNCH	DINNER
MON			
TUE			
WED			
THU			
FRI			
SAT			
SUN			

The path to healing begins with self-compassion. Be kind to yourself as you navigate this journey

Date:
....

Shopping List

Note:

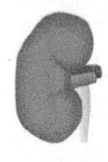

KIDNEY DIET
Meal Planner

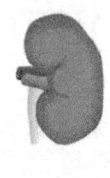

	BREAKFAST	LUNCH	DINNER
MON			
TUE			
WED			
THU			
FRI			
SAT			
SUN			

Patience is your greatest ally. Healing takes time, but every day brings you closer to your goals.

Date:
....

Shopping List

Note:

KIDNEY DIET
Meal Planner

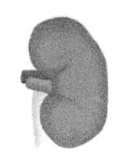

	BREAKFAST	LUNCH	DINNER
MON			
TUE			
WED			
THU			
FRI			
SAT			
SUN			

Surround yourself with positivity and people who believe in your ability to overcome. Together, you are unstoppable

Date:
....

Shopping List

Note:

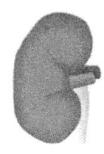

KIDNEY DIET
Meal Planner

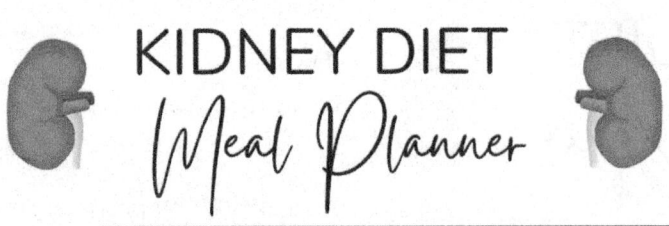

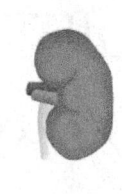

	BREAKFAST	LUNCH	DINNER
MON			
TUE			
WED			
THU			
FRI			
SAT			
SUN			

The journey to wellness may be long, but remember, you have the strength to make it.

Date: ....

Shopping List

Note:

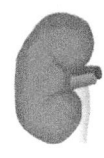

KIDNEY DIET
Meal Planner

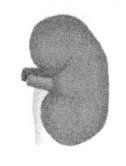

Date:

Shopping List

	BREAKFAST	LUNCH	DINNER
MON			
TUE			
WED			
THU			
FRI			
SAT			
SUN			

Hope is the heartbeat of resilience. Keep it alive, and you can conquer any obstacle.

Note:

KIDNEY DIET
Meal Planner

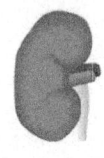

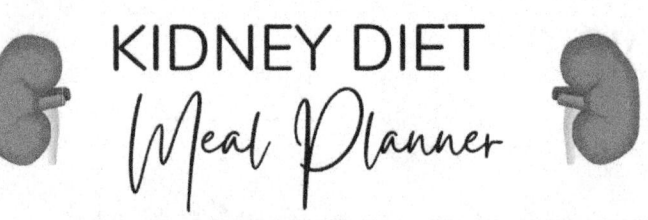

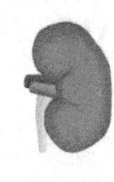

	BREAKFAST	LUNCH	DINNER
MON			
TUE			
WED			
THU			
FRI			
SAT			
SUN			

Your body is an incredible masterpiece. It has the power to heal and recover with the right care and love.

Date:
....

Shopping List

Note:

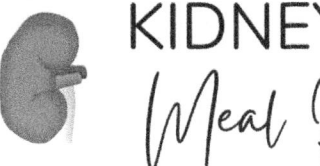

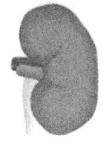

KIDNEY DIET
Meal Planner

	BREAKFAST	LUNCH	DINNER
MON			
TUE			
WED			
THU			
FRI			
SAT			
SUN			

You are not defined by your diagnosis; you are defined by your courage and determination

Date:
....

Shopping List

Note:

KIDNEY DIET
Meal Planner

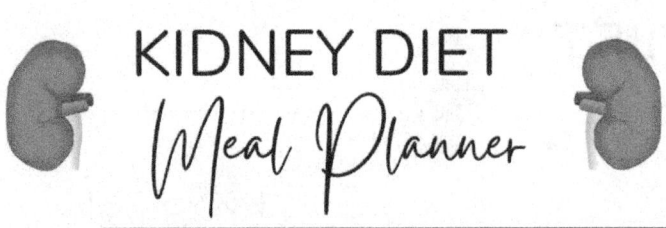

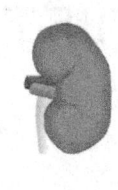

	BREAKFAST	LUNCH	DINNER
MON			
TUE			
WED			
THU			
FRI			
SAT			
SUN			

Small steps can lead to significant changes. Each healthy choice you make brings you closer to wellness.

Date:
....

Shopping List

Note:

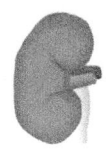

KIDNEY DIET
Meal Planner

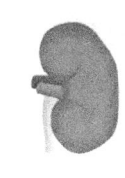

	BREAKFAST	LUNCH	DINNER
MON			
TUE			
WED			
THU			
FRI			
SAT			
SUN			

You are stronger than you know, and your spirit is more resilient than any challenge. Keep fighting, and never lose hope.

Date:
....

Shopping List

Note:

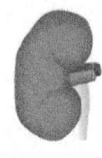

KIDNEY DIET
Meal Planner

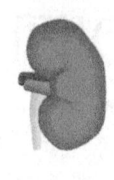

	BREAKFAST	LUNCH	DINNER
MON			
TUE			
WED			
THU			
FRI			
SAT			
SUN			

In the journey of life, challenges like kidney disease are just detours. Keep moving forward; your destination is worth the fight

Date:
....

Shopping List

Note:

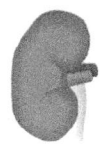

KIDNEY DIET
Meal Planner

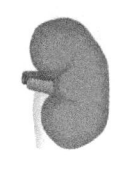

	BREAKFAST	LUNCH	DINNER
MON			
TUE			
WED			
THU			
FRI			
SAT			
SUN			

Your health is your most precious asset. Treat it with love, care, and the right nutrition.

Date:

Shopping List

Note:

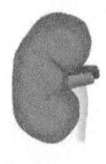

KIDNEY DIET
Meal Planner

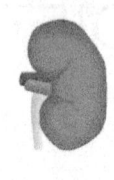

	BREAKFAST	LUNCH	DINNER
MON			
TUE			
WED			
THU			
FRI			
SAT			
SUN			

Believe in your inner strength; it's the fuel that keeps you going even when the road gets tough.

Date:
....

Shopping List

Note:

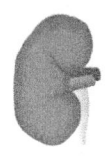

KIDNEY DIET
Meal Planner

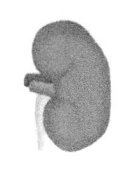

	BREAKFAST	LUNCH	DINNER
MON			
TUE			
WED			
THU			
FRI			
SAT			
SUN			

Every meal is a chance to nourish your body and nurture your kidneys. Embrace each bite as a step towards better health.

Date:

Shopping List

Note:

Made in the USA
Coppell, TX
14 June 2024